Praise for Debra Gaffney...

As Debra Gaffney's office manager I was honored to be an integral part of her practice the first six years of the AcuSET treatments. Her concern for patient care is absolutely primary. Debra welcomes each new patient and explains every step of her procedures. It was so exciting to witness the healing process! Her success is phenomenal! Many extremely allergic young children come to her clinic; they have not been off antibiotics since birth. These little ones are so subdued. Progressively, you can see that they are behaving like normal children: playful and alert. Many adults with debilitating diagnoses such as fibromyalgia are also so improved that they are back to golf and tennis again! Needless to say, Debra Gaffney's treatments come highly recommended! —S.O.

I have been treated by a medical doctor for rosacea. They told me there is no cure and gave me a lot of expensive creams, some that burned my skin. After the AcuSET treatment for my feather pillows I noticed a lot less redness in my face. I also had a problem with wool clothing. To me, wool always felt like steel wool in my hand. I could never understand why people would choose to wear anything that harsh on their skin. After the AcuSET treatments I can wear wool and it feels so much softer. —M.P.

I had lots of trouble with black peppers and red wine. After the AcuSET treatments, I don't. —B.W.

What are you willing to invest in improving your health?

While you might assume this is a question about money, it's not. It is a challenge to encourage you in gaining the greatest benefit from your treatment with Debra Gaffney and her staff.

This book provides you with a number of things you will find valuable. It:

- *outlines* the history of the treatment protocols used so you can know how and why they work
- *explains* the treatment program so you can know how to best plan your time
- *delivers* important information on how to receive the most from your treatments
- *de-mystifies* what might otherwise be a puzzling experience
- *recounts* patient histories to awaken and inspire you to the wonderful improvements that are very likely in store for you

No matter what condition brought you to seek treatment, no matter which protocol or protocols are applied, the information provided here will support you in taking maximum advantage of the relief that awaits you. With it, you may be able to activate your healing more quickly, and take it to deeper levels.

Coming in for treatment was a giant step in moving toward improved health and happiness. Take another by investing yourself in your treatment and reading what Debra has prepared for you.

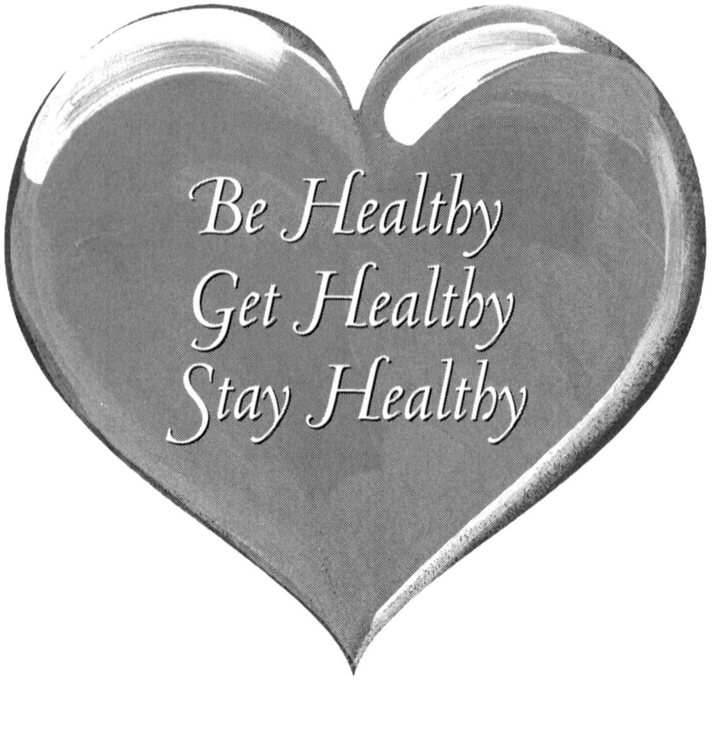

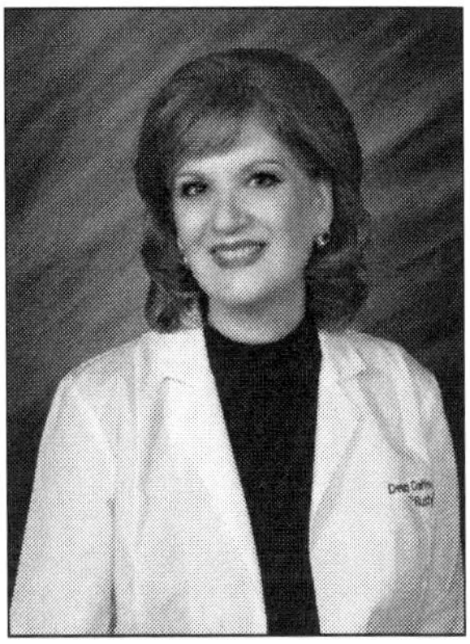

Debra "Rusty" Gaffney, A.P., C.C.P.A., has been involved with the healing arts since 1990. As a result of her extensive training and experience with Oriental Medicine, Acupuncture, nutrition, homeopathy and herbology, she has developed a highly effective protocol for neutralizing sensitivities that she has named AcuSET(SM). Since its inception in 2002, AcuSET has helped thousands of Debra's patients regain happy, normal lives. Debra has other degrees and certifications including a Diplomate in Acupuncture from the National Certification Commission for Acupuncture and Oriental Medicine and is a certified Chiropractic Physician Assistant. She has continually completed many other courses and post-graduate work.

When she's not seeing patients Debra spends her time taking classes and courses in her fields and enjoys reading, gardening, making jewelry, and playing with her two dogs and two cats. She and her husband, Dr. John Gaffney, a Chiropractic Physician, have lived in DeLand, Florida. for seventeen happy years.

Sensitivities

The Subtle Cause of Suffering,
the Hidden Cause of Illness

Serenity Pass Press
339 E New York Ave
DeLand, Florida 32724

SERENITY PASS PRESS
DELAND. FLORIDA

The field of Acupuncture and the treatment of allergies and sensitivities and nutrition are constantly changing. The author has taken great care in writing truthfully her understanding of the above health care modalities. The author always recommends her patients keep open lines of communication with their other health care practitioners. At no time does the author recommend her patients quit taking their prescription drugs without the knowledge of their prescribing doctors.

This publication is designed to educate and provide general information regarding the subject matter covered. It is not intended to replace the counsel of other professional advisors. The reader is encouraged to consult with his or her own advisors regarding specific situations. While the author has taken reasonable precautions in the preparation of this book and believes the facts presented within the book are accurate, neither the publisher nor author assumes any responsibility for errors or omissions. The author and publisher specifically disclaim any liability resulting from the use or application of the information contained in this book. The information within this book is not intended to serve as emotional or therapeutic advice related to individual situations.

Publisher's Cataloguing-in-Publication

Gaffney, Debra P.

Sensitivities : the subtle cause of suffering, the hidden cause of illness / Debra Gaffney. — 1st ed. — Deland, Fla. : Serenity Pass Press, 2008.

p. ; cm.

ISBN: 978-0-9801824-0-8

"Healing protocols for ending your discomfort and putting you on the read to health and happiness"—Cover.

Includes bibliographical references and index.

1. Allergy—Alternative treatment. 2. Food allergy—Alternative treatment. 3. Acupuncture. 4. Health. I. Title.

RC588.A47 G34 2008 2007909708
616.97/06—dc22 0802

Book Consultant and Shepherd: Ellen Reid www.bookshep.com
Cover and Interior design: Ghislain Viau
Photo of author: Fogelman Studios
Cover Photo: Art Lickey

Sensitivities

The Subtle Cause of Suffering, the Hidden Cause of Illness

Healing protocols for ending your discomfort and putting you on the road to health and happiness

Debra Gaffney A.P.

SERENITY PASS PRESS
DELAND, FLORIDA

Contents

Acknowledgements I

Chapter 1: How AcuSET℠ Came to Be 5

Chapter 2: The Methods Behind AcuSET 17
What Is Acupuncture? 23
Balance 24
Qi 25
Blood 27
Yin and Yang 27
Acupuncture Terms 29

Chapter 3: Defining the Problem 39
Items That Contain Corn 42
Items That Contain Eggs 42
Items That Contain Milk 43
Items That Contain Formaldehyde 43
Symptoms of Sensitivities 43
Anxiety 45
Arthritis 46
Asthma 50
Constipation 57
Coughs 58
Diarrhea 59

Digestive Problems 62
Fibromyalgia 64

Chapter 4: Office Visits 69
Your First Visit 69
Your Second Visit 74

Chapter 5: About Our Treatments 77
Vials 81
Needles 81
Cupping and Gua Sha 83
Moxabustion 86

Chapter 6: Your Treatment 89
Planning Ahead 90
Appointment Scheduling 91
Instructions for the Treatments 91
Before You Leave Your House 92
At the Clinic 92
Toxicity and Detoxifying Treatments 93
Order of Treatments 93
At Home 127
What Happens If… 127
Trying a Treated Item 128
Anaphylactic Shock 128
Missed Appointments 129

Chapter 7: Testimonials 131
Pain 132
Palpitations 135

Anxiety 137
Fibromyalgia 138
Digestive Problems 140
Headaches 141
Cough 143
Sinus Conditions 144
Skin Rashes 145
Hearing Problems 147
Sneezing 147
Pediatrics 149

Chapter 8: More Information 157
Supplements 159
Vitamin A 165
B Complex 166
Vitamin B2 (Riboflavin) 167
Vitamin B3 (Niacin, Nicotinic Acid and Niacinamide) 167
Vitamin B5 (Pantothenic Acid) 168
Vitamin B6 (Pyridoxine) 169
Folic Acid 170
Vitamin B12 (Cobalamin) 170
Biotin 172
Vitamin C 172
Vitamin D (D3) 173
Vitamin E (Alpha, Beta, Gamma, Tocopherol) 174
Vitamin K 174
Calcium 175

Magnesium 176
Iron 176
Potassium 177
Proteins 178
Fats 179
Carbohydrates 180
Fiber 181
Enzymes 181
Oriental Nutrition 182
The Five Energies of Food 182
The Five Flavors of Food 186
Movement of Food 189
Common Organ-Related Ailments 191
Ailment-Specific Foods 192
Foods to Help Correct Symptoms 196
Herbal Medicines 198
Homeopathic Medicines 201
Laughter 203
Tension Releasers 203
Breathing Techniques 204
Exercise 205
The Best Diet 206

Treatment Schedule 211

Bibliography 215

Index 221

Acknowledgements

I thank my wonderful husband, number one mentor, and biggest supporter, John Gaffney, D.C. He helped me create this book, saw more in me than I ever saw, and pushed me to achieve the confidence to dedicate my life to helping sick people get healthy.

I thank Dr. Peter Fernandez, who encouraged me to write this book and for introducing me to the best book shepherd around, Ellen Reid. I truly thank all the wonderfully patient team members in getting this book together. It was fun having "people" guiding and making this book make sense!

I extend my gratitude to Denise Heist for teaching me how to use the computer, typing my manuscript, and finding the correct spelling for all those "strange words." I want to thank my best friends: Johanna Gulliver for reading the manuscript, helping me keep it readable, and showing me how to type in colors on the computer; Buffy Williams for her encouragement and e-mails and beautiful affirmations; Jonathan Ellis for support during this process; and Rev. Nancy Saputro for keeping me on the right track.

Of course, I also thank my mom and dad, Elizabeth and Jim Pardee; my sister, Michele, for her support and encouragement; and my brother-in-law, Warren, who kept me laughing during this time. I thank my brother and all my other relatives for encouraging me in all I do.

Thanks to my excellent teachers at the School of Complementary Medicine as well as my "study buddy" in school and Oriental Medicine mentor, Dr. James Kim. I also thank Dr. Ellen Cutler and Dr. Devi Nambudripad for developing the techniques that saved my life. I know I would have not made it this far without NAET and BioSET and in turn my patients also thank them.

Most of all, I thank my patients. Hundreds of them participated in the case histories and testimonials. They had faith in me and followed my suggestions and kept my spirits up while we worked on their problems and turned them into healthy people.

I wrote this book as an aid for my patients. Anyone can read this book and come away with an understanding of Acupuncture and alternative health care. I hope you share this information with family, friends, and your medical doctors. Some of the things you read in this book you will find hard to believe. Every day my staff and I see results that are amazing.

There are quite a few testimonials included. My patients have enjoyed reading them through the years and have told me these testimonials have encouraged them to try this technique. I have put my heart, soul, blood, sweat, tears, and Qi in this book and in my practice. It distresses me to see people of any age suffer needlessly. If you're not sure if we can help you, I BEG you to ask us. Eighty-five percent of all my patients have been helped and are satisfied. The remaining fifteen percent weren't completely satisfied and I continue to try to find a way to help them. There are no guarantees in life or medicine, but this technique cannot hurt you in any way. The only side effects are healthy, wonderful side effects!

And lastly, thanks to my coworkers (especially Rose, our office manager and boss) who daily helped me make copies, find books, files, bragged about the book to everyone, and encouraged me.

Chapter 1

How AcuSET Came to Be

While I was studying at the School of Complementary Medicine, a classmate asked me to treat her with a new technique for sensitivities. She said that she would hold a vial of a herbal medicine a teacher had prescribed to help her sleep. The problem was that the medicine made her sick. She asked me to insert needles in specific Acupoints. After that treatment, she would need to be away from the substance for twenty-four hours, but after that she would no longer be sensitive to the medicine.

Well, of course, I thought she was crazy! But my classmate had read about Nambudripad's Allergy Elimination Techniques or NAET, a means of eliminating allergies that involved a variety of medical philosophies including Acupuncture, nutrition, allopathies and others. She always knew about the latest and greatest in health care techniques and liked to try new things. I on the other hand was very skeptical about most everything, including a lot of the information I received at school on Acupuncture and herbal medicines. Still, I did what she asked to humor her. Two days later, she said that she could take the medicine without any side effects.

That same week, my husband, Dr. John Gaffney, had a patient approach him with the same request. This patient had a book describing the treatment for sensitivities. Doc shared the experience with me and we read the book that night. We weren't sure the technique was worth the effort; it seemed far out.

Still, I thought about my classmate and Doc's patient all night. In a strange way, the concept made sense. The next day, I asked Doc to treat me for MSG.

I had avoided this additive at all costs. It was not easy going to an Oriental Medicine school and not eating Chinese food! When I was just fifteen, Chinese food put me into the hospital for the first time. I had become sick before we had even left the restaurant. While I was attending the Oriental Medicine school, I rarely ate out because I could never be sure if the food had MSG in it.

My reaction to anything with any derivative of MSG was horrendous. It would start about twenty minutes after

I ate. My face would get numb. I would suffer with a blinding debilitating headache for twenty-four hours. I would have projectile vomiting for hours. I would have to lie in bed in a dark room, my whole body aching so much I could hardly move. At the end of twenty-four hours, I would be exhausted and usually stayed in bed another day.

In fact, the last time I had had MSG (under a different name in vegetarian sausage), I could have died if Doc had not been there to help me.

During that night after we talked about the treatment, I kept thinking how limited my life was becoming. We traveled a lot to conferences and classes. I took food with me to eat on the plane and at the hotels. Would I take this chance or forget about it? Even now, nine years later, I remember the calmness I felt the next morning. I was sure I was going to do this!

I went to the grocery store and bought pure MSG. That night, Doc treated me. Forty-eight hours later, I went to a Chinese restaurant twenty minutes from my house. I took along a girlfriend in case something went wrong. I ate everything—soup, egg rolls, dark gravy, hot spices, and the dessert.

Nothing happened at all, no numbness, dizziness, or anything.

At this same time, Doc had a blood test to identify allergies. His joint pain had grown worse; after thirty years of running three miles per day, he couldn't run anymore. At the end of the day, his feet would be purple, painful, and hot. A blood test showed that he was allergic to twenty-five items out of fifty. He started doing the elimination and rotation diet, in which all known foods to which you are allergic are eliminated and one of those foods is reintroduced every three days. Doc had to avoid most fruits and grains.

The next week, we went to an internal disorders conference. At least five doctors came up to us and asked if we had heard of Nambudripad's Allergy Elimination Techniques or NAET. It is named for Dr. Devi Nambudripad, who had created the treatment almost fifteen years earlier.

The other doctors all said it changed their lives, their families' lives, and their patients' lives. At the end of the weekend, Doc convinced me to attend the classes. I was waiting for my license to practice Acupuncture and had some free time. In addition, he knew that once I found something that interested me I was like a bulldog with a meaty bone. The next available class was two months away.

During this time, I treated Doc with Acupuncture for some of the foods his blood test rated as high. One day, I treated him for wheat and, after I ate a sandwich I kissed him. We noticed that his stomach instantly started to swell. That night he said he felt like he had meningitis; every joint in his body hurt.

My first NAET class looked like a cross between a Mary Kay convention and a revival. More than a hundred people were there to see Dr. Ellen Cutler, who was teaching the course. Long lines formed to buy Dr. Cutler's latest book and buy vials. It was hard to find a seat. We were scrunched in like sardines all three days. Some people stood; some sat on the floor till they could get more chairs. There was a great feeling of excitement in the room, and that feeling stayed all weekend. Doctors who used the technique were sharing their experiences. One doctor in Georgia had a seven-month waiting list. The classes went till ten each night, but no one seemed tired.

Dr. Cutler, who once was a patient of Dr. Nambudripad's, had developed BioEnergetic Sensitivity and Enzyme Therapy, or BioSET, which includes computerized electrodermal screening (EDS). Dr. Cutler was using muscle testing, which involves exposing muscles to possible allergens to check people for sensitivities. I have a problem with muscle testing because it can be subjective, you can only test for a few items, and it is hard on both parties. Dr. Cutler then showed us the computerized equipment and software program.

Dr. Cutler tested me and said I was very sensitive to eggs. I told her eggs never bothered me, but she suggested I go home and get treated for eggs and call her. Doc treated me, and the next morning I woke up without a stiff neck for the first time since I was a teenager. I had always joked I had married a chiropractor for that reason! I have not had that stiff neck in the nine years since the treatment.

I bought the program and started treating Doc and other family and friends, and Doc treated me.

We treated Doc for twenty-five of the fifty items his blood work had identified. After the treatment, those items were fine, but the items for which he was not treated remained positive. His blood work showed reactions to fruits such as bananas and cantaloupe as well as grains and beef. I had those reactions and many more, including wool. I was surprised; I had thought I was sensitive only to MSG.

After using Dr. Cutler's technique, I developed AcuSET. Here's the background on how AcuSET came to be.

I wanted to reduce the number of patient visits; other practitioners were treating patients for forty to sixty visits, at great expense to them. Also, the strategy of requiring patients to avoid for twenty-five hours the items Dr. Cutler used was difficult at best. I had undergone the procedures and found that it could be impossible to avoid some of the items I was allergic to for even one hour.

Occasionally, there were side effects, such as headaches, nausea, and tiredness if the patient was exposed to the items in that twenty-five-hour time period. I also hesitated to encourage my patients to fast because Oriental Medicine does not recommend it. And, if someone had low blood sugar, fasting would be out of the question.

Some of my patients came to Florida from out of state and had to stay in hotels for one to two weeks. For some, this was great as they were away from their pets, their dust and mold, and their gardens. However, they also could be exposed to things that could trigger a reaction such as old smoke, cleaners, dust, and mold that were different from the items at home.

Most patients could tolerate two treatments in sixteen hours; some could handle three. We had to be careful not to combine in a single day certain treatments such as meat and grains. I was not inclined to treat some of my weakest patients with certain items due to the stress it could create for them and because of possible failure of the treatment. It was very complicated to choose the items to treat in that time frame without putting a patient on a fast.

Most of my patients were in an extremely weakened state and needed to eat every few hours. But, for example, if we treated a patient for B vitamin complex and later on for hormones, all he or she could eat for thirty-six hours were peaches. I tried it myself and could do no more than sit in a chair for most of the day.

There were so many treatment items that were difficult to avoid. For instance, how can anyone avoid cotton for a whole day? One of my patients did. She wore only silk and sat on leather or plastic for twenty-five hours, which was not an easy feat! She had to stay out of rooms with drapes and could not use a towel to dry off. This woman was desperate and was very pleased with the results, but was not looking forward to another day like that one.

Occasionally, unpleasant side effects such as headaches, coughing, sneezing, tiredness, depression, or itching occurred. These symptoms would usually last no more than four hours. Still, if it happened to you, it wasn't pleasant.

I knew there had to be a simpler way. The patients' side effects sent me back to the Oriental Medicine books.

The body has twelve Meridians or pathways, each of which is most active for two hours of the day. I wondered if reactions were due to an item upsetting a particular Meridian. My patients were a determined bunch and viewed these reactions as proof that something was happening and were eager to go on. I knew I was dealing with an incredible modality, but it needed to be easier and more affordable.

After one year of research; trials and errors; taking classes; researching books on Acupuncture, physiology, nutrition, allergies, homeopathy, and psychology; and working with my husband, I decided to slowly add more than one or two vials of like materials per treatment. I tested the vials separately and together on the EDS machine (*see Chapter 5*) and recorded the reactions. Then I treated with those vials using my new Acupuncture protocol. I kept adding vials and mixing different categories to a point of saturation. Two weeks after the treatment, I would retest. If the treatment held and symptoms were diminishing, I would continue.

The next problem was the avoidance time. It was almost impossible to avoid most substances for twenty-five hours, and some items could not be treated at all. I continued to use different Acupuncture points, adjusting the number of needles and use of the electro-Acupuncture machine.

The technique that resulted is AcuSET. It's not a cure-all, but it can have a huge positive impact on your life and health. My patients tell me how wonderful it is to cut their grass and not be sick the rest of the weekend, or to go to work and not become ill because a coworker wore perfume that day, or to bring home a puppy and have your asthmatic child not react at all. I have treated over a thousand people with better than an eighty-five percent success rate. I have put my heart, soul, blood, sweat, tears, and Qi into this book and into my practice.

It distresses me to see people of any age suffer needlessly. My typical patient is a woman between forty and seventy years old. She has suffered for years with myriad problems, takes four to six medications a day, and can't remember the last time she felt good. She is almost always overweight, and this baffles her. She wakes up planning her next nap. She works and has a family. We are her last resort. Men usually come to us when their spouse is tired of their snoring or lack of energy.

We also have a large pediatric practice (*see Chapter 8*). Children respond quickly to AcuSET.

In the last thirty years, medicine has changed very dramatically in our country. When I was in grade school, only one child in class was overweight. One had asthma and one had allergies. We never heard the phrases "learning disabled" or "ADD." We ate lunch brought from home and we played outside. We rarely went to a doctor. We went to bed at night and slept all night. We never ate in a fast-food restaurant. We were healthy and happy.

Now, I talk to teachers who tell me children are always out sick or attending school sick, which spreads the "sick-ness." The school nurse hands out medicine prescribed by doctors. I see children in my office who have been sick since they were born. Their moms always say the same thing: " When you get him/her better I'll come to see you for the allergies I've had since childhood. Do you think it's heredity?"

If you're not sure if we can help you, I BEG you to ask us. There are no guarantees in life or medicine, but this technique cannot hurt you in any way. The only side effects are wonderful—more energy; a general sense of better well-being; and an end to sneezing, runny noses, joint pains, rashes, headaches, and bowel problems.

Chapter 2

The Methods Behind AcuSET

Over five thousand years ago, Chinese doctors were trying to find better ways to treat their patients. These doctors were very observant as they had little else to work with. A doctor would study his patients by looking at the color of their skin and eyes as well as their teeth and gums and tongue. The doctor would also touch the patients. They would be feeling for tightness, looseness, lumps, heat and cold.

Questions were asked about every aspect of the patients' lifestyle. Were cool days enjoyable or did the patients huddle by the fire? When it rained, did they feel their aches more? What happened when it was windy? What did their bowel movements, urine, vomit, and so on look like? Did heat feel better or did it make them uncomfortable? What food did they enjoy eating and which foods made them sick?

Nothing was left unasked. At the regional gatherings, the doctors would compare notes. Symptoms were categorized; conditions were examined. Did the patients in the southern part experience the same conditions as patients in the north? The patient who had fallen off a roof would tell his doctor that it felt better or worse when his wife rubbed his back. Some doctors tried using a flat stone and pressing down on the patients' spine. It felt good; in fact, if the stone was heated it felt better.

The doctors also discussed what worked and didn't work in herbal medicines. Health care did not "just happen" but was experimented with for thousands of years.

Fast-forward to a few thousand years later (approximately 2000 B.C.) and doctors still were getting together to learn from each other about techniques and instruments. Much experimenting was done on prisoners and family members of the doctors. "Lines" could be traced along the body, and tenderness or tightness would be felt. Doctors began using bamboo and bone rather than stone for needles; these would actually go into the sore spots and relieve pain. When these new needles were inserted, sometimes the pain would go away. If not, then other "points" or "lines" were used. In 1760 B.C. during the Shang dynasty, bronze was used in manufacturing needles; gold and silver came about in 500 B.C.; and in 200 B.C., steel was created.

~ Chapter 2 ~
The Methods Behind AcuSET

Sometime between 300 B.C. and 100 B.C. Ch'I Po wrote *The Huang Di Nei Ching Su Wen,* which contained detailed descriptions of pathology, treatment plans, anatomy, and physiology. It talked about Yin and Yang (*see page 37*) and described organs and diseases of the body. The Nei Ching talked about 160 points for needling the body to foster healing. It described different needling techniques and nine different needles. Translations of this book are still studied today.

During the sixteenth century, the physician Li Shi Shen wrote fifty volumes of a book called *Ben Cao Gang Nu* (Material Medica). It discussed uses for over fifteen hundred herbs and contained ten thousand herbal prescriptions. He also established the pulse positions acupuncturists use today. Several other countries (Japan, Korea, India, and Pakistan) were also using Acupuncture at this time.

Acupuncture in the United States came with the migration of the Chinese in the nineteenth century. Those adventurous enough to see a practitioner in San Francisco at that time would have been examined and treated in almost the very same way we examine and treat today. Why mess with something that works? Acupuncture helps the body heal itself. Acupuncture treats the body as a whole and not just a body of parts.

Acupuncture had an earlier and more visible exposure in Europe than in America. A Dutch doctor, W. Ten Rhyne (or Willem Ten Rhijne as some books spell his name), in 1683 wrote the earliest published European report on Acupuncture. He also studied in Japan where a Dutch company employed him as its physician.

In France in 1735, a group of Jesuit priests wrote about Acupuncture and the Chinese method of diagnosing after visiting China. One technique I use came from these books. A hundred years later, Acupuncture was used for treating patients in Europe. The conditions treated were neuralgia and rheumatism. It spread to England, Germany, and Italy.

After the late nineteenth century, most European doctors were not practicing Asian medicine, instead using needles to explore tumors or for local pain relief. Medicine was changing rapidly, and homeopathy (which has its roots much earlier) was in vogue.

We did not see Acupuncture used in Europe again until the 1950s. At that time, it was used across Europe as well as in Russia and the Middle East. Most of the Acupuncture research outside of Asia has been done in France and Germany.

Recent U.S. interest in Acupuncture began in 1972 while President Nixon was on a trip to China. One of the reporters covering the trip, James Reston, suffered an appendicitis attack. After surgery, Acupuncture was used to control his pain. Reston wrote about it in *The New York Times.* Doctors in the United States were fascinated by Acupuncture and started hiring doctors from China or went to China to learn.

In the last ten years the United States has been doing research. Acupuncture and research can be found in most teaching hospitals such as Shands at the University of Florida in Gainesville and all Mayo clinics. The National Institutes of Health (NIH) is conducting fifty-four different Acupuncture studies. One of my Asian teachers asked why the American people would not accept Acupuncture until they researched it for "years" when Asia had done over five thousand years of constant research. A good "point."

Today, you can't pick up a magazine without reading an article on Acupuncture—it's on the television almost weekly somewhere. Even Oprah tried it on TV—live.

Most people sense that there must be a better way to achieve and maintain health. After all, their parents and grandparents did just fine and rarely took pills or saw a doctor. Why are we so sickly and dependent on drugs when we live in a time with all the technology for safeguards to ensure healthy food, water, and air? Why do we not know how to get healthy and stay that way?

Why is Acupuncture popular in the United States now? It works. People are tired of a health care system that does not look at them as people but as hearts, lungs, or joints—and diseased ones at that, without any hope for health. People are tired of taking pills that cause other problems and send them to yet another doctor for more pills.

What Is Acupuncture?

The easiest way to understand Acupuncture and Oriental Medicine is to visualize yourself as a Christmas tree with fourteen strands of lights. Some of your light bulbs are blinking nicely. Some are blinking fast; some are dull; and some aren't blinking at all. These light bulbs are your Acupuncture points.

The electrical wires of the strand of lights are the Meridians (pathways/channels) and the current running through the "wires" is Qi (energy). The Meridians are translated into English and are named as organ systems. They are Lung, Large Intestine, Stomach, Spleen, Heart, Small Intestine, Bladder, Kidney, Pericardium, Triple Warmer, Gall Bladder, and Liver. Meridians work with more than the organs named. For example, the Lung Meridian deals with respiratory tissues and skin; the Kidney Meridian handles problems with the kidneys as well as hair, teeth, joints and many other functions in the body. There are two other Meridians called Ren and Du.

The Meridians start on your feet and hands, travel up, down, and around your body. Two Meridians, the conception vessel (Ren) and governing vessel (Du), run up the front and down the back connecting around your mouth and anus. (AcuSET does not involve needling around private parts, in the mouth, or close to the eyes.)

For example, each ear has over 160 points that correspond to body parts and systems. There is really a complete body in each ear. A procedure called ariculotherapy involves the shallow insertion of tiny needles into the external ear. I have always felt that using this procedure created a more thorough treatment. There are some incredible calming points on the ear and I use them at every treatment.

Each Meridian except the Ren and Du Meridians has its own flavor, color, sound, time of day, season, and emotion. There are strong and weak times of day. As we listen to you and examine you, we can decide which Meridian needs treatment. Your skin color gives us information, as does your emotional state. The colors are red, green, yellow, white, and blue (black). There are faint colorings throughout the face. Some people have dark circles under their eyes, and some people have red noses. We are trained to look at the whole face for different colors. These colors correspond to different Meridians. We see this in your face, feet, and hands. Different colors on different parts of your face tell us volumes! Certain conditions have an odor. For example, bad breath tells us the Stomach Meridian is out of balance.

Every Meridian has a pulse (except Ren and Du)—six on each wrist, three deep and three on the surface. I mentally place each pulse in one of twenty-eight degrees or categories to help me identify the situation. I will check them periodically to determine whether you are accepting the treatment.

Balance

If there were one word to describe Acupuncture and Oriental Medicine it would be balance. Every action or nonaction by our body (in and out) has one important function: to balance us. This is called homeostasis.

The ancient Chinese knew that humans and the earth are nature. What hurts one hurts the other; what heals one heals the other. The energy that flows through the body is similar to a river carrying energy. We suffer the same conditions the earth does—too much dampness, dryness, wind, cold, or heat.

When we have balance in our life, everything is better. We're happy; we feel alive. We have the energy to do what we want and need to do. Our emotions also crave balance. Lifestyle changes, exercise, sleep, food, and water all help us to achieve this elusive balance. The ancient Chinese understood and wrote about this thousands of years ago. The world hasn't changed much since then, has it?

Now, you are changing it for yourself. You started by reading this book and making your first appointment for Acupuncture. Any time in the future when you feel "out of balance," call your Acupuncture physician. The Chinese felt it was important to get a treatment at least every time the seasons changed. That's every three months. Most of your cells renew themselves every three months. Coincidence? I don't think so.

Qi

Qi (pronounced chee) should be the easiest thing to write about because it is everything and everywhere. The best way to describe Qi would be to say it is "energy," except that Qi is much more than energy. When we have enough Qi we feel good. We feel alive, are active, sleep well, think well, and everything seems to be going our way. When Qi is deficient, we wake up tired—if we were lucky enough to get to sleep. We don't want to eat—or we eat everything in sight, mostly the wrong foods. We might crave certain foods like those with sugar or salt.

We can't see Qi, but we see the results of Qi. Look at nature; you don't see the wind, but you do see the branches and leaves moving. You see water moving down a stream. Did you ever wonder what is moving the water? It is Qi.

In our bodies there are different types of Qi. We are born with Qi that we inherit from our parents. This is a very good reason to be in the best health possible before you conceive a child. This is called Original Qi and needs to last us through our lifetime. We get Gu Qi through our food, drink, and the air we breathe. Qi is in each cell and organ.

The body takes Qi from the food and drink we ingest and transforms and transports it through the body to be used as Qi and Blood. When Qi flows in the right direction we are fine, but if it reverses flow we cough, hiccup, or vomit.

Qi moves freely throughout bodies except when we are not healthy, when it gets stagnated. This tells us there is a blockage and the Qi needs to be moved. It can be felt as stabbing pain.

Each Meridian has its own Qi. For example when we breathe, the Lung Meridian grabs the air and sends it through the correct pathways where the Kidney Qi will pick it up. The Kidney Qi then separates the pure from the impure, and urine and carbon dioxide are formed. Urine is excreted through the kidneys and bladder, and carbon dioxide is expelled through exhaling.

As I've said, Meridians run along our bodies like strands of Christmas tree lights. At certain "points" there is a difference in the energy's electrical aspect. These places are called Acupoints. When needles are inserted in these specific spots, Qi can be moved, strengthened, or unblocked.

Qi is quite magnificent. As you receive treatments, you will learn to feel and identify Qi. You want to do all you can to increase your Qi. Eliminating your sensitivities is a very good first step!

Blood

When we talk about your Blood in my office, we are not talking about your blood that you see when you get cut. We're talking about Blood as a form of Qi moving through your veins. Blood causes Qi to move with it. If you have pain that doesn't move from one area to another and is stabbing in nature, we say you have Blood stagnation. If you feel weak or dizzy; have pale skin and lips; are losing your hair; and have dry skin, you are most likely suffering from Blood deficiency. We can build our Blood with Acupuncture, food, herbs, and rest. Qi and Blood move and work together and need to be nourished to do this work.

Yin and Yang

You are probably familiar with the terms Yin and Yang and have seen the Tai Ji symbol. It is the circle colored half black with a white dot and half white with a black dot. There is a little Yin in Yang and a little Yang in Yin as in ALL things.

In the darkest of night comes a bit of light with the sun peeping over the horizon. Everyone has experienced "blinding light," a light so bright you can't see anything. Cold can be so cold it feels hot and burns. This means there is a constant changing aspect to all things. This changing keeps all things in balance. For example, women have a lot of female hormones with a little bit of male hormones. Men have a lot of male hormones with a little bit of female hormones.

Yin represents the female, cold, nighttime, moon, inside, interior, front, Blood, bones, moistness, solid, softness, static, deficient. Yang means all the opposites; heat, daytime, sun, outside, exterior, back, Qi, skin, dryness, hollow, hardness, movement, and excess.

This brings us back to *BALANCE.*

Acupuncture Terms

Blood (Xue): The Oriental explanation of Blood differs from the Western explanation of Blood. In the Oriental philosophy, Blood is the densest fluid substance in the body; it is a form of Qi. Blood gives nourishment and supports our body. Blood moistens skin, hair, tongue, eyes, and sinews. Blood helps to anchor the mind and calms the emotions. If someone can't sleep we say the mind floats. Blood is stored by the Liver, generated by the Spleen, governed by the Heart and is the mother of Qi.

Cold: Are you colder than the people around you? Cold problems are characterized by aversion to cold, desire for heat, hypoactivity, lack of thirst, loose stool, paleness, lethargy, dullness, weakness, large amounts of clear urine, thick odorless discharges or phlegm usually white in color, pain, cramps, and spasms. A "Cold" condition is treated differently from a "Hot" condition.

Damp Heat: This is a condition of dampness and heat that occurs in the Large Intestine (diarrhea with mucus and blood), Bladder (urinary tract infections, kidney stones), and Gall Bladder (gallstones).

Dampness: Can also be living in a damp house or a physical condition. Dampness in the body usually appears during damp and humid weather. Symptoms are feelings of heaviness in the head and limbs, swelling, bloating of chest and abdomen, edema, nodular masses, watery stool, sore joints, large amounts of sticky discharges, phlegm, and lethargy.

Deficiency: A lack of Qi or Blood or a result of weakened function of the organs or Meridians. Over time, a deficiency can become physical and emotional symptoms and signs, which are considered "normal" health problems.

Deqi: Translates as "arriving of Qi"—the feeling of obtaining the Qi with the needle, which the patient may experience as a slight pressure, fullness, numbness or a tingling sensation. These sensations are normal and let the Acupuncture physician know that the treatment is working. This is the "product" of major research across the world since the early 1950s. Books written as early as AD 652 talk about Deqi.

Disharmony: Lack of harmony and balance in the body due to the stagnation or imbalance of Qi. This can be caused by physical or emotional trauma, environmental factors, or an excess or deficient condition.

Disperse. A needling technique that moves, circulates, and distributes Qi to relieve the stagnation of Qi and Blood, or the accumulation of Heat, Cold, Dampness or Phlegm.

Distal Points. Acupuncture points that are away from the area of pain or disease. For example, we can use a point on the hand for a toothache rather than needling the cheek.

Dryness. Affects the fluids of the body. Symptoms may include dry skin, chapped lips, dry cough, dry mouth, dry eyes, and constipation.

Eight Principle Patterns. Signs and symptoms have a deeper meaning in Oriental Medicine. We look at patterns to find the cause; this helps us to organize diagnostic information according to the principles of Yin, Yang, Interior, Exterior, Hot, Cold, Excess, and Deficiency.

Excess: When Qi, Blood, Phlegm, urine, sweat and tears are out of balance and accumulate, leading to symptoms and signs of an abundant nature.

External Factor: External factors are Cold, Damp, Wind, Dryness, and Heat and can affect the body.

Essence (Jing): The material basis of an individual's life. It starts with our parents. It is stored in our Kidneys and is fluid like Qi. It is very precious and must not be squandered by excess alcohol, sex, poor diet, overwork, lack of rest, or a wild lifestyle.

Food and Environmental Sensitivity Assessment: This is a computerized electrodermal screening that helps to identify your body's response to certain foods and items you may come in contact with. See Chapter 5 for more information.

Holistic: The word comes from the Greek "holos," meaning whole. Holistic medicine involves all areas of your life. We don't just treat your indigestion, but all the other symptoms. We treat with a philosophy that includes a comprehensive and complete agenda to heal your mind and body through exercise, diet, Acupuncture, Chiropractic, reflexology, and massage.

Homeostasis: The ability of the body to maintain sameness. Homo means man, stasis means same. The body does this by adjusting physiological processes, despite constant varying external conditions.

Heat: Illness caused by heat is demonstrated by constipation, dehydration, fever, hyperactivity, inflammation, swelling, skin rashes, restlessness, agitation, insomnia, scanty dark urine, and strange-smelling body secretions.

Internal Factors: Any factors affecting the body that come from the inside of the body. This is usually due to an imbalance or disharmony of Meridian and organ systems.

Imbalance: Lack of balance that leads to stagnation, weakness, or excess of Qi and our internal environment. This will lead to illness, disease, and pain.

Meridian Stress Assessment: A computerized electrodermal screening program that will help us determine the start of your Meridians (pathways). It will show us which Meridians are on the low side or high side pertaining to energy. You will get a printed computerized diagram. In addition, we will take your pulse measurements manually.

Meridians: Also called Channels. These are pathways in which the vital energy called Qi circulates through the entire body. Meridians are connected to every organ system. There are fourteen main Meridians and many other channels.

Organ Systems: The Five Organ Systems—Liver/Gall Bladder (Wood), Heart/Small Intestines (Fire), Spleen/Stomach (Earth), Lung/Large Intestines (Metal), and Kidney/Bladder (Water)—organize all physical and mental processes and join together all of the structural components of Meridians, cells, tissues, muscles, and organs. Each Organ System is connected to a Meridian. Together, they do everything that needs to be done in our body.

Pathogen: An external factor such as bacteria, virus, or fungus that can cause illness, disease, and pain.

Phlegm: Comes after dense, congealed dampness that can cause cysts, obstructions, mucus, nodules, lumps, or tumors. It can be yellow, white, red, clear, or brown.

Qi: The pictograph or Chinese character of Qi means "vapor," "steam," "gas," and uncooked "rice." It can be as immaterial as vapor or as material as rice.

Sedation: Two conditions excess in the body under physical stress. An Excess or a Deficient condition. Excess must be calmed down, or "sedated," with needles or herbs.

Seven Emotions: Throughout life we experience many different emotions, some more than others. When these emotions are repressed, hidden, erratic, or excess, it can lead to disease and illness. These emotions correspond with a Meridian. The seven emotions–shock and joy (Heart); anger (Liver); fear (Kidney); sadness (Lung); worry and pensiveness (Spleen/Stomach).

Spirit (Shen): Refers to the mind and emotions. How you view life and relate to others. We can see it in your face and your eyes and hear it in your voice and your speech.

Stagnation: What happens when Qi and Blood don't move. It is pain or bruising.

Tonify: An Acupuncture needling technique used to nourish, supplement, support, and invigorate your body through the Meridians and Qi. To "Tonify" is to add to the body's vital energies to restore and promote homeostasis of the organ systems.

Traditional Chinese Medicine (TCM): An ancient and complete holistic system of health care that has been around for more than three thousand years. It includes Acupuncture, herbs, Oriental nutrition, movement, and balancing the Qi and Blood to bring the body back to homeostasis.

Wind: A Wind illness affects the lungs, throat, head and skin, and is demonstrated by aversion to drafts, spasms, pains that move from body part to body part (a very key clue to diagnosing), dizziness, vertigo, trembling, itching, headache, stuffy nose, scratchy throat and numbness. These symptoms occur suddenly. When you suffer from "the common cold," an Acupuncture physician will diagnose it as one type or the other. The two types are "Wind Heat" with a sore throat and fever or "Wind Cold" without a sore throat but with sniffles, runny nose, and sneezing.

Yang: One of the two forces that organize the universe and all in it. Yang manifests as fire, heat, restlessness, dry, hard, daytime, sun, energy, expansion, light, time, activity, and male birth. See this chapter for more information.

Yang Organs: Known as the "hollow organs" that transform matter, transport and store body substances and discharge waste. The Yang Organs are the Gallbladder, Small Intestine, Stomach, Large Intestine, and Urinary Bladder.

Yin: One of the two forces that organize the universe. Yin manifests as moon, shade, rest, earth, female, blood, solid, soft, darkness, quietness, cold, inertia and death. See this chapter for more information.

Yin Organs: Known as the "solid organs" that store the Essences of the body. The Yin Organs are the Liver, Heart, Spleen, Lung and Kidney.

Chapter 3

Defining the Problem

Some reports state that sixty percent of adults suffer from food sensitivities. Some experts say food sensitivities have increased over thirty-five percent in the last twenty years. Food allergies are less common and are identified by a blood test or a scratch test on the skin. You do not need a blood or skin scratch test to tell you that you reacted in a negative way to something you ate recently or used in preparing a meal.

Food sensitivities can manifest in many different ways with many different ailments. They are reactions to a food eaten, smelled, or touched. People with food sensitivities feel like they are classic hypochondriacs. Some react if they get within inches of a particular item. Some complain of feeling bloated or of puffiness around the eyes and nose. This could be the body's confused overactive immune system surrounding the cells with a watery substance to flush away the invaders (normally harmless items). Cells get waterlogged and tissues swell. Hands, ankles, and feet can swell. Another common reaction is sneezing and a runny nose. I have had patients who have a constant runny nose when they eat. Others experience rapid heartbeats or drowsiness. It's not unusual to experience symptoms and not link them to sensitivities.

What causes food sensitivities? Well, people eat more wheat, corn, milk, and eggs than ever before. If we look at the typical diet, we see an increase in fast foods, restaurant foods, and commercially prepared foods. These foods usually have extra fat, fillers, additives, and chemicals in them. Studies prove that these food items show most of the reactions and symptoms.

How are we going to digest and assimilate genetically altered food? Not too well, I'm sure. When human bodies "showed up" over two million years or so ago, they expected to eat naturally occurring foods. We ate fruit, vegetables, nuts, fish and nonbeef meats. Milk and wheat were not introduced into the human diet until ten thousand years ago. Sugar wasn't eaten much till the 1900s.

We have evolved and adapted, but not quickly enough to handle the food changes in the last thirty years. When I started studying nutrition in the seventies, it was estimated we each ate fifty pounds of sugar a year; today, the number is 135 pounds per person, quite an increase.

You can look around and see the evidence. We have five immunoglobulins in our blood serum. They are similar and different. They protect us from invaders such as viruses, bacteria, and allergic reactions. When our body thinks something strange has invaded, it goes into attack mode and eventually creates antibodies against the invaders. The invaders can be bacteria, viruses, a food, or chemical; the antibodies are protein molecules or immunoglobulins.

Our body starts to protect us at birth. Food allergy symptoms generally don't occur immediately (except in the case of anaphylactic reactions) due to the release of the IgE to the cells. This can take up to three days from the exposure. This is because the IgG antibodies are circulating. IgE and IgG are different types of protein molecules that register allergic responses.

Food cravings also are a common sensitivity symptom. People complain of being "addicted" to certain foods. I have a patient who ate a dozen eggs a day. Guess what? That was her number one sensitivity. Another patient ate handfuls of salt every day; her number one sensitivity was salt. Brain chemicals are released and cause a good feeling when you eat the offending food. When you quit eating it, you have uncomfortable to strong reactions, so your brain tells you to eat it again.

It's hard to avoid items you are sensitive to as they are in almost everything we eat or touch or smell. Here are just a few examples:

Items That Contain Corn

Aspirin and tablets such as vitamin or over-the-counter drugs unless stated to be corn-free, baking mixes, powdered batter mixes, breads, cakes, candy, catsup, some processed cheese mixes, cookies, corn cereal, corn meal, corn oil, popcorn, doughnuts, corn starch, cough syrups, baked goods, salad dressings, corn chips, taco chips, crackers, gravies, grits, chewing gum, gum or adhesives, glue, ice creams, jellies and jams, some liquors, processed meats, peanut butters, powdered sugar, puddings, some salts in containers for smooth flowing, processed sauces, soups, syrups, toothpaste, and body powders.

Items That Contain Eggs

Bread, bread crumbs processed for frying, cake mixes, french toast, cakes, some pie crusts and cream pies, meringues, ice cream, sauces, meatloaf, noodles, pancake and waffle mixes, puddings, and soups.

Items That Contain Milk

Bread mixes, baked goods, prepared sauces, cheese, chocolate, batter for frying mixes, gravies, soups, pancakes, waffles, ice cream, cream desserts, and processed potato dishes.

Items That Contain Formaldehyde

Rat poison, fertilizers, disinfecting materials, antiperspirants, dyes, carpets, furniture, insecticides, clothing, nail polish, embalming fluids, and makeup.

Symptoms of Sensitivities

If you suffer from any of the following symptoms you might have sensitivities:

Anxiety
Arthritis pain
Asthma
Back pain
Blood pressure (high or low)
Breast lumps
Breathing problems
Cold/flu
Constipation
Coughs
Cramps
Cravings
Depression
Diarrhea
Digestive problems
Dizziness
Eyes dry/red
Fatigue
Headaches

- Hot flashes
- Incontinence
- Indigestion/gas
- Insomnia
- Joint pains
- Lack of energy
- Migraines
- Nausea
- Neck pain
- Night sweats
- Overeating
- Painful menses
- Palpitations
- PMS
- Rashes/acne
- Sore throats
- Toothaches

For example, it is not unusual for someone to come in to our clinic with a complaint of migraines that occur every week. I had a man who suffered like this every day. He would vomit at night for hours, which would stop the headaches till the next morning. Another patient suffered like this, alternating between vomiting and migraine headaches, for more than twenty years.

I believe we develop sensitivities because we don't have a correctly working digestive system with the right enzymes to process our food. Whole natural foods have those enzymes to digest themselves but processing kills them.

For example, after age forty, we produce less hydrochloric acid. A symptom of this is heartburn or an acid taste. People think they have too much acid when this happens, but the opposite is true. They will then take an antacid and their problems become worse.

Other digestive factors are eating too much at one time, eating under stress, being under stress, not chewing correctly, drinking too many liquids with meals, drinking cold or iced liquids, and eating too many cold or raw foods. In the Oriental Medicine way of thinking, studying during meals pulls the Spleen Qi away from its job of transporting nutrients. Mealtime needs to be a calm and relaxing time to enjoy your food without cell phones, work, or unpleasant conversation.

Patients have almost always seen their physician for the symptoms above and have a diagnosis with proper medication. I will clarify how Oriental Medicine explains some of these symptoms and how AcuSET treats them.

Anxiety

Anxiety causes panic attacks, shakiness, palpitations, racing heart, hyperventilation, dizziness, headaches, diarrhea, vomiting, unexplained fears, feelings of dread, and insomnia. Sufferers can't calm down, and have a feeling of lack of control over their life. In Oriental Medicine, this pattern of symptoms is usually connected to the Heart, Liver, and Kidney Meridians.

Anxiety also involves deficiency of Qi, Blood, Yin, and Yang. The most common causes of anxiety are sensitivities to food colorings and additives, sugar, alcohol, and vitamin B complex. After sensitivities are eliminated, I find that people who complain of anxiety are calmer and sleep better. We also instruct on breathing techniques, exercise, and proper diet to help improve lifestyles.

Arthritis

Arthritis pain is the second most common diagnosis we see in our clinic. I was surprised to learn that sensitivities could cause pain and inflammation.

In Oriental Medicine, joints are the place where Qi and Blood gather. When heat, cold, dampness, and wind attack it causes a painful obstruction syndrome. There are two types of this condition and they are called "Bi Syndromes". One is called a "Cold Bi Syndrome" and the other is called a "Hot Bi Syndrome." The patient usually knows if their joint pain feels hot or cold to them. Another way to tell the difference is if heat feels good on the joint, it is the "cold" type. In Western Medicine it is classified as wear and tear on joints and degeneration of articular cartilages such as knee, hip, ankle, wrist, and finger joints. As time goes by, there can be pain, stiffness, and inflammation.

My husband had been a runner for thirty-five years without any problems. One day, he showed me his feet;

they were almost purple and felt very hot to my touch. He complained of pain, something he never did!

He told me that he suspected allergies to bananas and wheat were causing these symptoms. I thought he was crazy, but he made an appointment for allergy tests. The tests came back with twenty-five out of the fifty items tested for as moderately severe allergies.

I was still not sure about the connection between the arthritis pain and moderately severe food allergies, but agreed not to feed him those twenty-five items. And they were good foods, not junk foods!

After a couple of weeks, he was a little better but not enough to make either of us happy. I started buying bananas again; I figured I didn't have arthritis pain so I could eat them. His symptoms got worse! This was about the time I learned about NAET and we decided to try it on both of us *(see Chapter 1 for more details)*.

We also continued to treat Doc for the foods on his list, and he gradually got better. Three months later we tested him on the computerized electrodermal screening equipment. The items that we had treated him for were at zero, meaning no reaction to them; the items for which we had not treated him were still reactive. In the next two weeks we treated Doc for everything from previous blood testing lists and new items we identified from the electrodermal screenings. That was eight years ago. He hasn't had pain since then.

There are different types of arthritis: rheumatoid; lupus; and osteoarthritis, which is the kind I just described. I have treated patients with all three types in various degrees of pain and inflammation with good to excellent results.

One of my patients could not drive, dress herself, shop, clean house, or cook due to rheumatoid arthritis. She spent most of the day sitting in a chair. All day long, her pain level would be ten—unbearable—on a scale of one to ten. She was on seven medications and was very depressed. We had difficulty getting her up on the table but she insisted on lying down for the treatments. She would curl up almost in the fetal position as she could not lie straight. I treated her with Acupuncture for two weeks. She noticed a little pain relief, but was still in a very bad state.

I told her what I had done for my husband. She said she had nothing to lose, so we tested her for food sensitivities. She had quite a number of them and her reaction numbers were quite high. We proceeded to see her two times a week for the next three weeks. The Friday after Thanksgiving, she called me at home and told me she had done dishes for the first time in twenty-five years. "I'll see you on Monday," she said, "and I might drive myself." When

I saw her, her fingers weren't as curled as they had been and she was on less pain medicine, but more importantly, she felt more like a person again.

Another woman who had been diagnosed with rheumatoid arthritis a few years earlier approached me after one of my lectures. She was in severe daily pain. She worked and cared for her family and tried to keep a workout schedule. She was on a lot of medication and was not happy with the side effects. I explained that we had had success with rheumatoid arthritis, but that we would need to examine and test her before determining if we could help. The next morning, she came in; my staff rearranged my morning appointments because it usually takes a week to get an appointment for testing. We found multiple sensitivities and started treatment that day. She started getting pain relief after a couple of weeks. I find that most people start to see results in two weeks. At the end of six weeks, she was very pleased.

One remarkable symptom about this lady was the intense heat coming from her fingers. I could actually feel it six inches from her hand. As time went on, the heat and the pain both decreased.

After the initial schedule of treatments, we both agreed that she needed to continue on a twice a month visit schedule for a few months. During this time, she had a previously scheduled appointment with her physician. She was able to show him greater range of motion and reduced swelling. She told him she was for the most part pain-free and that the heat in her hands was gone. He said he was glad the medicines worked; she told him she had quit taking them (I didn't know this) months earlier and was using Acupuncture. He was not pleased and told her she would come crawling back for her pain medications very soon. She hasn't, and it has been four years now. She comes to see me for treatment every other month for a "tune-up," and the first thing I check for is the heat in her hands. It has never come back!

Asthma

In Oriental Medicine, we use the term "asthmatic breathing." This is different from the medical diagnosis of asthma. A patient may have trouble breathing with some wheezing – this is asthmatic breathing. Clinical definitions of asthma indicate inflammation of the airways with coughing, chest tightness, and wheezing and trouble with inhaling and exhaling.

The Lung Meridian governs the function of breathing and protecting the skin. The Lung Meridian is easily affected by wind and cold, heat and dryness. When someone comes in with coughing and sneezing and with a weak voice we diagnose Lung Qi Deficiency or wind cold. If the person has these symptoms and a sore throat, we call it Lung Yin Deficiency or wind heat. These conditions are the common cold and flu. We can also treat these problems with Acupuncture.

"Asthmatic" patients have many more symptoms with greater severity than those with flus and colds. They cannot take in a breath or exhale. Unless you have experienced this disorder you cannot imagine the panic they feel. I have treated successfully many more asthmatic cases than the ones below. I never tell them to stop taking their medicines or inhalers. In fact, my first asthmatic patient still carries her inhaler at my insistence but has not used it in seven years!

One very chilly day in January two years ago, I walked into a treatment room to see my next patient. I instantly realized I did not know this patient and that she was having trouble breathing. I took her pulse and said that I needed to call 911. She said she wouldn't go if I did call 911 because they couldn't do much more with her. She had driven more than forty-five minutes by herself to get to my office. I quickly inserted needles for breathing problems and sat down next to her, knowing I'd be calling 911 in a few minutes. In about fifteen minutes, she started to breathe more normally. She told me that she was feeling less tightness in her chest and would be fine. We were able to do a full new patient evaluation and I listened to her story.

I had suffered from asthma and allergies for over sixty-five years. I had tried all the treatments that any allergist had. In January 2005, upon awakening I could not breathe. I realized I had a few minutes to reach my inhaler and get some air to my lungs. Finally, I could breathe but was faced with the problem of getting emergency help.

I was alone as my husband was out of town. Miracles happen. My phone rang and it was Debra Gaffney's office. I had been waiting for an appointment. I told them I could not come in as I was having a major asthma attack. The voice on the other end of the phone said, "We can take care of that." Within the hour I was there and Debra proceeded very cautiously to do Acupuncture on me. I was so ill I didn't mind that I had never had Acupuncture before.

About fifteen minutes later, I felt such relief. I had the feeling that that huge elephant had gotten off my chest finally! I could breathe! I had never had such relief that quickly before. Through testing I learned I was sensitive to some of the stuff I was taking to help my asthma.

I still see her sometimes as a new problem will come up and my lungs are still slightly weakened. I can now eat tomatoes and strawberries, go to homes that have dogs, cats and birds, walk every day, breathe the air, and do almost anything I could never do most of my life. I am a new person inside. I am no longer mentally confused. I think clearer; I feel healthier. I have no reflux problems, no allergies or asthma. I am thankful for this miraculous treatment of AcuSET and Debra Gaffney. They are an answer to my prayers!

In my first month of practice, a local doctor referred one of his asthmatic patients to me. This pleasant lady was a retired massage therapist and "wanted to do things in a more natural way." We conducted the Meridian Stress Assessment and Food and Environmental Sensitivity Assessment. Her Lung and Kidney Meridians were very weakened. The Spleen and Liver Meridians were in an excess state. She also complained of lots of phlegm, anxiety attacks, diarrhea, and stomach problems. I treated her for the next six months with remarkable results. The following year she moved out of state to be near family. She contacted us to say good-bye, and said her asthma was much better and that she didn't go to the emergency room very often.

My allergies seemed to come on very suddenly. I would be fine in the morning, then by the afternoon I would become ill. One time, I was put in the hospital with pneumonia. The first time this happened was when we were on vacation in New York. Then that evening on the way back to the hotel I started feeling very strange. By the time we arrived at the hotel, I just wanted to go to bed. A couple of hours later I woke up and told my husband that I thought maybe we should go to the hospital. The doctor asked me how long I had been sick. I told him that it was since that afternoon. He could not believe that anyone could be that bad in just a few hours. He wanted me to be put in the hospital immediately. I chose to fly back to Indiana and went to the hospital at home.

This went on for a few years. No one could find out what the problem was. The only treatment that would help at all would be IVs of antibiotics. Most of my hospital stays were from five to eight days. Before long, scars were showing up on my lung X-rays because I'd had pneumonia so often. They did constant blood tests to try to find out the cause and came up with nothing. After several severe bouts of pneumonia, I lost my sense of smell.

The pain of trying to breathe was so intense that a few times I prayed to just stop breathing.

I went to an allergist for testing. We did find out that I did not have asthma. That was about all we found out. Then one day quite by accident, we found a possible cause. We were with a group of people and one of the young girls had just put on perfume. When she came back and sat behind me, the coughing, wheezing, and shortness of breath started! It was so bad that we had to go to the emergency room. Then my husband noticed that whenever I was around perfume or aftershave or other scents, the reactions would start. Since I had lost my sense of smell, I could not tell when people had on scents. The allergy got so bad that I was housebound for almost four years.

During this time at home I had lots of time to get information from the Internet. I then came across the information about NAET. The more I found out about this treatment, the more encouraged I became. Then came the challenge of finding someone who could do the treatment. After talking with Rusty, I knew that she had that special gift. I first went to her on April 3, 2002. That was the day that my life changed!

I had treatments with Rusty for two months. The change in my life is nothing short of incredible. I have been able to go shopping and am actually regaining my sense of smell again. I tell everyone that they need to come to Rusty for treatment. It is just incredible to be able to be a person again. Life is wonderful. I am so thankful that Rusty has taken the time and effort to learn this technique and is willing to share her skills to make people well again. To think that something so easy and painless can give people a life free from all the suffering.

Strange things happened to some people after the hurricanes in Florida in 2004. They developed allergies and asthma for the first time. The only explanation I had was the presence of trees, weeds, flowers, and plants that were chewed up and spit in our face from other parts of the state. A few months later, I noticed a weed I had not seen before. I checked the "weed" book and found they came from a different part of the state. I developed a cough that was so severe I couldn't sleep. I carried this weed to our agriculture center for some advice. By the time the master gardener came out to see me, I couldn't talk at all! I went home, held that weed, and gave myself a treatment. The next day I was fine.

A woman who suffered greatly after the hurricanes and was on medicine for life was referred to me by a relative. Her CT scan showed problems in her lungs. She suffered with coughs, sinus pressure, chest tightness, breathing problems, and headaches. Ten days after her treatment started, she went off her medicines. Again, I do not encourage this and caution against it. She finished her course of treatment and one year later is fine. Another scan showed great improvement.

A gentleman from Wisconsin showed up on our doorstep for treatment of allergies and asthma. His dad had heard a woman at the post office telling another woman about our treatments. He was only going to be here a week or so. He kept an "Epi pen" on his belt because he could have a severe anaphylactic reaction at any time. I typically didn't take cases like his, but since he had come so far and promised not to ever eat anything that gave him a reaction, I agreed to treat him.

His test turned out not to be particularly unusual. We saw him twice a day for four days. He reported feeling fine and went back to Wisconsin. I called him a few months later, and he said he had not had one episode of asthma and no allergic reactions.

A friend of mine referred a woman to our clinic. This dear woman had asthma and sinus problems with so much phlegm that she couldn't walk near perfume or smoke without a severe episode. She rarely went to church and almost never could be in a place with smokers. After five treatments, she walked next to a man smoking and nothing happened! A week later, she was in a kitchen that became filled with smoke and nothing happened. Everyone was amazed! She was still having trouble with perfumes in church, so we concentrated on fixing the remaining problems. Two months later, she was able to stay in church and even went back for an evening recital.

Constipation

Not all constipation problems are from food sensitivities; a lot are from lack of adequate fluid intake, fiber, and exercise. Oriental Medicine explains constipation as Heat in the Large Intestine or a Dry Large Intestine. If there is pain, mucus, and blood, that would be Heat obstructing the Large Intestine and on the level of irritable bowel syndrome.

We can treat all types of bowel disorders with Acupuncture. If a patient comes in with sinus problems and constipation we schedule him or her for testing with the computerized electrodermal screening equipment and Food and Environmental Sensitivity Assessment. Sinus problems are also covered under the Large Intestine Meridian.

An elderly gentleman came to see us. His daughter said that he ate a lot of pasta and rarely ate fruit. He had not had a bowel movement in seven days, no matter what they did to help it move along. He felt fruit caused him gastric distress although there was no medical confirmation for it. I treated him for the sensitivities to fruit and asked if they were going straight home. His daughter assured me they would. Two hours later, I got a phone call from her. They had decided to stop at a Chinese restaurant for lunch, and he had had four bowel movements before the cookies arrived as a result of the AcuSET treatment.

Coughs

One delightful woman was a smoker and coughed all day long for ten years. Her lungs were fine, according to her medical doctor. The doctor said there was no cancer or emphysema, she had a cough left over from a cold. She was given different allergy medicines with very little help.

The cough bothered her, her family, and coworkers. Her husband could not hear the TV when she was around.

She was desperate and decided to give Acupuncture a try after a friend told her we had helped with her cough.

We did the usual MSA and FESA testing and determined that her Lung and Kidney Meridians were in a weakened state. Her Liver Meridian was excess as was her Stomach Meridian. This also produced phlegm. These findings were consistent with Oriental Medicine and we proceeded to treat her. Within a few weeks, her coughing was subsiding. After a month, her coworkers asked her what she was taking for her cough. Six weeks after treatment, she played eighteen holes of golf without coughing. She also quit buying allergy medicine. We continued to see her once a month for a year. I ran into her in the store recently and she reported she was still not coughing but would really like to come in for tune-ups to keep healthy.

Diarrhea

Diarrhea, ulcerative colitis, and irritable bowel syndrome are three entirely different problems in Western medicine. In Oriental Medicine, they are in the same ballpark. Diarrhea is watery or loose stools. This can be caused by something in the diet, a virus, traveling to a different country with contaminated water or food, food intolerance, poor food handling and storage, or a plain old flu. Ulcerative colitis is a chronic disease that typically involves blood in the stool with severe pain and weight loss. Irritable bowel syndrome can have bouts of constipation and diarrhea. Sometimes there is mucus in the stool. When there is constipation, the stools can be hard like marbles.

When we examine and diagnose in the Oriental Medicine model, we ask questions that are strange to some people. I need to know if your stool smells or floats, what color it is, whether your rectum burns before or after you evacuate, and the time of day you evacuate. These questions help us determine the Meridians involved so we can better treat you.

Diarrhea with pain means the Liver Meridian is involved or there is Heat in a Meridian. A bad odor also means Heat. Without odor, the problem could be Cold in a Meridian and a diagnosis of Spleen or Kidney Yang Deficiency. If the stool is followed by blood, the Spleen Meridian is involved. Very dark stools mean Blood Stasis; bright red blood means Damp Heat in the Intestines. I've included a testimonial from a friend and two other stories.

This woman's experience is not as unusual as many may think:

> *Have you ever had dinner and five minutes later had to run to the bathroom because you knew you were going to have diarrhea? Have you ever had abdominal cramps that were as bad as labor*

pains and made you cry? Have you ever been afraid to put anything in your stomach because you knew you would have diarrhea?

Well, I have experienced all of the above and more. It is like having a constant, horrible stomach virus. I have suffered from irritable bowel syndrome on a steady basis for the last eleven-plus years. Prior to that time I would have occasional bouts of diarrhea, not knowing why or where they came from. They would last from an hour to a day or so, sometimes one or two times a week. I sometimes could go a week or more without any cramps or diarrhea.

In 1998, I had a very severe episode that lasted about four days. I missed work; I had drop-to-my-knees abdominal pain, and could not be away from a bathroom. In ten days' time I lost nearly thirteen pounds that I could not afford to lose. By the time I was able to see someone for a colonoscopy some seven weeks after the severe episode, my colon was still quite irritated and inflamed. That surprised the doctor. During that seven weeks I had eaten only rice, applesauce, and baked potatoes. I continued this diet at least a month after the procedure and lost more weight.

During this time, I still had severe stomach cramps that medication controlled somewhat but did not eliminate. I took a prescription to stop the diarrhea on a daily basis. After the colonoscopy, I was told by the surgeon not to eat any dairy products, red meat, salads or raw vegetables, anything with any kind of cream sauce or spices, or anything greasy or fried. So, I was very limited in my food choices. I improved somewhat, but still had diarrhea on a regular basis—sometimes daily, sometimes four to five times a week, sometimes up to eight or ten times a day, but seldom fewer than three or four times a day. That continued until I began Acupuncture. In all I have had three colonoscopies, taken up to eight doses of my prescription drug (my limit) a day to stop the diarrhea, and taken medications that did not really help my irritable bowel.

Since I have had the Acupuncture sensitivity treatments, I can eat almost anything. To me, that is a major accomplishment after years of worrying about when and/or where the bouts would hit me. I feel better; I'm surely not as tired. I am not stressed about leaving the house because I might have diarrhea, and my insides do not hurt from going to the bathroom all the time.

Amid the Acupuncture treatments for the colon and sinus, I showed a few symptoms of a cold several different times, but a few sneezes and a couple days of a running nose were all that ever developed. I never had such a slight cold before; in the past, a cold could put me down for days.

Digestive Problems

In Oriental Medicine, the Stomach and Spleen Meridians transform and transport the food and nutrients. The Stomach Meridian "cooks" the food; the Spleen Meridian separates the "essences" from the food and drink, then transports the pure essences to the Lung and Heart Meridians where they become Qi and Blood. We try to educate our patients on the correct eating habits (*see Chapter 9*). If you came to us with the medical diagnosis of GERD, you may be given a diagnosis of Stomach Yin Deficiency or Stomach Fire.

We have treated patients who just feel queasy after eating to patients who vomit most days. One young woman was very pale, thin, and tired. She vomited daily. She had no emotional problems and was not bulimic. She had gone through psychological counseling for vomiting and taken many medicines. We tested her and found many, many sensitivities. After one week of treatment, she was able to keep food down. Three weeks later, she came in for a treatment and told me she had eaten at a restaurant and went to an amusement park and rode a roller coaster with no problems.

I was plagued for months with a digestive/elimination problem that my gastroenterologist could not treat. He told me to write down everything I ate, figure out what foods caused the problem, and simply NOT eat them anymore. Meanwhile, I'd heard about Debra Gaffney from several individuals including a chiropractor and a neighbor. My neighbor claimed Debra Gaffney had cured her of her asthma. "HUH? How could that be? How could Acupuncture cure anyone of asthma?" was my reaction.

Then, in March 2005, for two days I felt as if my whole digestive system was suffering the consequences of eating the hottest, spiciest Mexican food available. Out of desperation, I called Debra Gaffney's office and made an appointment for the next day.

When I got there, I started reading through the AcuSET procedural paperwork that her assistant gave me. I almost walked out. I was stunned and overwhelmed with what looked like an impossible bunch of pre- and post-treatment protocols to follow. However, since I was already there, I stayed and went through my first Acupuncture treatment with her. I followed her post-treatment rules and went home.

The next morning, the burning sensation in my digestive tract was gone. My bowel activity was completely back to normal. During the six-week treatment process, I realized that I was actually tasting food subtleties again. I wasn't bruising the way I used to (for example, if I even thought about running into the coffee table, I would bruise). A podiatrist had told me the plantar fascitis on my right heel would never completely heal, and that I would have to wear arch supports for the rest of my life. Suddenly, it was gone and has yet to return.

Fibromyalgia

Fibromyalgia has many different painful, uncomfortable symptoms including but not limited to sleep problems; headaches; sensitivities to light, smells, and sound;

numbness; tingling feelings in hands and feet; a sense of hopelessness; and depression. There is also an incredible feeling of exhaustion. The pains can be dull, shooting, stabbing, burning, and deep, or the skin can be sensitive to touch. Other symptoms include restless leg syndrome, mood swings, night sweats, shortness of breath, bladder problems, jaw pain, skin rashes, blurred vision, swollen feet (day and night), dizziness, cold hands and feet, a fast heartbeat at times, chemical sensitivities, and allergies.

We see a lot of patients with fibromyalgia and have a very high success rate. We may have to treat them with only Acupuncture for a couple of weeks if they are in a weakened state. If that's the case, we then do the computerized electrodermal screening and begin the AcuSET treatments. After we have cleared sensitivities to vitamins and minerals, we prescribe the correct nutritional supplements. Most patients are fifty percent better in a few weeks. It's not unusual for them to go back to work full time with a renewed interest in life.

Many years ago, I worked for a chiropractic physician in Connecticut. Our office was near that of an allergy specialist who would send patients to our office for care. These patients were almost "bubble people." They could not live any type of normal life and went to great lengths to get well or at least a little better. They would go on very restrictive diets to the point of eating only one item for four days at a time. One patient could only wear white cotton. One patient could not use electricity.

One day, I stood by the file cabinet and prayed with so much feeling that there must be a better way to help these people. About that same time a woman was seeing this doctor. Here is her testimonial.

Allergies have ruled my life since puberty. By age thirty-seven, I was fighting fatigue, pain, and truly severe anxiety attacks, one of which kept me hiding under the bed for two days. I became suicidal.

A famous allergy doctor diagnosed the problems and hospitalized me in Zion, Illinois, in an environmentally controlled facility. During the three-week hospitalization, I was detoxed by four days of total fasting and then tested for food and environmental allergies. The testing showed I was able to tolerate eleven foods and had many environmental allergies. I had to avoid fluorescent lighting, natural gas, and all petrol items. I lived on mono-food meals (one of which was steamed onions) in a four-day rotation, wore only cotton, and carried a charcoal mask to avoid environmental fumes. It sounds bad, but I was pain free and had no anxiety attacks.

I was still plagued with times of sudden weakness, and the formaldehyde fumes were lessened but not eliminated. At the age of fifty, a viral infection damaged the left ventricle of my heart, lowered the ejection rate to twenty-nine percent, and caused arrhythmias.

Now a new round of allergies began as side effects to prescription drugs. These manifested as anxiety attacks, arthritis, fibromyalgia, fatigue, weak legs, and many other symptoms. Meanwhile the food and environmental allergies were again a problem.

At age sixty, I began Acupuncture with Debra Gaffney. Now, at sixty-six, I have an ejection rate of forty-five percent; use no prescription drugs; am free of pain, fatigue, and anxiety attacks; and am able to enjoy many more foods. I am truly grateful to Debra Gaffney for her knowledge, her skill, and dedication.

A seventy-year-old woman with an endless list of symptoms came to us as a direct referral from a chiropractic physician. She had been diagnosed with fibromyalgia in 1978 and was desperate for something to work. She rarely slept and when she did, had strange dreams. She bruised easily, suffered with sinus problems, and had daily headaches. She had pain over her entire body. She broke out in rashes if she took any medicines. Her appearance and dress was immaculate. She did nothing all day except try to get through her days. She had tried Acupuncture in California and felt it had helped.

On testing with the EDS, we found the health of her Meridians was very poor. I could barely find a pulse on her, certainly not twelve of them! Her test scores were very high especially on heavy metals and chemicals. She wanted to be treated more than the usual twelve visits because her pain level and tiredness was so severe she couldn't do anything anyway. So we saw her three times a week for three months and then once a week with good results. Over time, her symptoms decreased in severity and number and she was quite pleased.

Chapter Four

Office Visits

Your First Visit

Oriental Medicine and Acupuncture have an individualistic and complex approach to diagnosis and treatment. In my practice, you will be examined and treated as a whole body, not just a gall bladder or back pain.

Before you meet me, you will be asked to complete an extensive health questionnaire. Feel free to bring lists of medicines, vitamins, herbs, surgeries, test results from other physicians you have seen.

I will review your questionnaire (intake form) before I meet with you. As I walk into the room, I will observe your skin color. Is it red, pale, tinged with yellow, dark around the eyes, gray around the mouth?

Then I will listen. This is your time to tell me everything that concerns you about your condition. You are not complaining but explaining. I want to hear your story in your own words. As you talk, I will listen to the sound of your voice, the strength of your voice, and your breathing. I will notice how you sit, if you rub sore areas as you talk, how you get up and move around.

Next you will be shown to a treatment room that is not too cold or too hot. It will have a comfortable table and soft music. Here you will remove your shoes and socks and be asked to lie on your back. You will rest here for a few minutes, hopefully relaxing a little.

I will then check your pulses, six on each wrist. This will give me a better idea of your health. Your pulse diagnosis is very valuable. This technique goes back at least two thousand years and is based on the principle that Qi and Blood move through the body as one. Feeling the pulses is a learned art; a bad pulse is weak, very slow, slippery, and tight. A good pulse is even, strong, and smooth.

I place me hands on each wrist, gently press down a fraction of an inch, then let up and feel the pulses on the surface. I feel the blood coursing through the veins like anyone else taking your pulse but we know that your Qi is the moving force of the blood. I am feeling the strength, rate, rhythm, size, and harmony. I'm looking for excess and deficiency. If the pulse feels like it is pounding and trying to jump out of your skin I say it's excess. If I can barely feel it, it's deficient. There are further quality and degree separations.

I give you a chart with your pulses on it, and we can discuss it at length. I review your pulses on each visit. This is how I can tell you're improving even if your symptoms are clearing out slowly. I can tell if you are tired, had too much caffeine, or had a cigarette recently. I have taken postgraduate classes and read over ten books on the subject.

This is a strange concept to anyone in the Western world who has taken pulses on patients in a hospital or doctor's office. I was one of those people. After checking pulses on thirty patients one morning, I KNEW there were twelve pulses! The hard part is interpreting them.

One teacher told me that the Chinese practitioners feel you can't really know how to interpret a pulse until you have done it for twenty-seven years! Hopefully, in another sixteen years, I will be "really" good at it! I check pulses two to three times during a treatment.

When patients leave, their pulses are much better than when they came in. On patients who come in at least every three months, I can feel an improvement that doesn't diminish very much unless they "come down with something" or have a major health challenge.

On a pregnant woman we can feel a quality that resembles someone having two pulses inside. We call it slippery. Not the same slippery as someone with a cold, though. It feels like running your fingers over a dish of pearls.

Another aspect of diagnosing is looking at your tongue. The appearance of your tongue gives a good indication of the health of your organs. Your tongue can change its appearance daily. It can have white gooey stuff on it, or it can be any shade of yellow to brown. It can have scalloped edges; a raw tip; swollen, thin, dry, moist quivers; or any combination of the above. If it is short, we know there is a cold condition going on; too long, there is heat.

The tongue is a map to the body. The Heart is on the tip and the Kidney is in the back, Lungs on the sides with

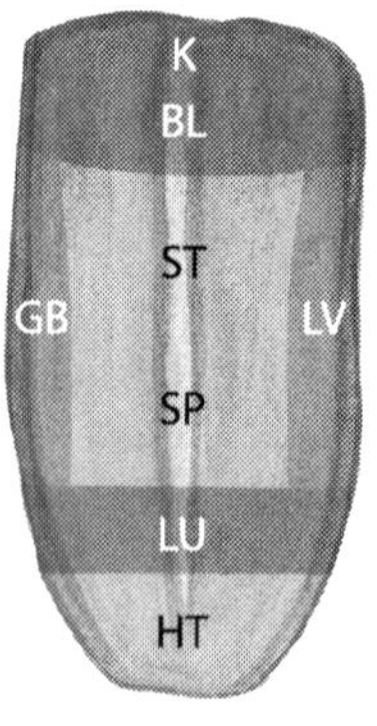

the Liver and Gall Bladder. The Stomach and Spleen are behind the Heart in the middle. Some tongues look raw; some are dark red or pale. There is so much information on your tongue!

After gathering information, I am ready to treat you. I will then wipe off twelve or so spots (Acupoints) with alcohol and insert needles. Usually they are inserted only a fraction of an inch. The usual placement of needles is on your hands, arms, legs, and feet. Maybe one will be placed between your eyebrows for relaxation and a few in your ear. These needles are solid, not hollow like hypodermic needles. They are flexible and as skinny as hair. They may have a plastic colored handle to indicate size.

You could feel a little sting like a mosquito bite when the needles are inserted. Rarely does this cause pain, but be sure to let someone know if there is pain after the needles are in your skin.

I will then check your pulses again and leave the room. It will be peaceful and dimly lit. If you wish, you may be covered with a special blanket that will not touch the needles. Always let the staff know what you need to be comfortable. You will usually be here for twenty to thirty minutes. Your pulses determine how long your treatment will be. The pulses will be checked during the treatment and will change for the better.

When I decide your treatment is finished, I will remove the needles by giving them a little pull or twist. It may happen so fast you won't see it.

At this point you and I decide if you are a candidate for the AcuSET treatments. If so, I will explain the computerized testing. An appointment will be made for the next available testing day, usually within a week.

If your pain is related to an injury, we won't proceed with the treatments unless there are secondary symptoms that are sensitivity/allergy related. If you are in a very weakened state, we may use Acupuncture for a few weeks to strengthen you and then do the AcuSET treatments. This happens perhaps ten percent of the time.

Your Second Visit

Your second visit will be the actual testing appointment to determine if, what, and how many sensitivities are affecting you. As we proceed with the testing, you may ask questions, although sitting back and relaxing is good too. We can stop and take a break if you need to and drinking water is encouraged. This is the electrodermal computerized screening test. We refer to it as EDS or Food and Environmental Sensitivity Assessment (FESA).

When the test is completed—usually after about a half hour—you will be directed to a treatment room similar to the one used for your first visit. When I join you, I will explain your test findings and the approximate number of visits needed to correct the sensitivities. Together we will review the symptoms that brought you to our clinic. The Acupuncture treatment will be similar as the one you received on the first visit, but this time treatment vials will be introduced. The vials are in a glass jar with a lid on it that will be placed near you. You don't have to hold them; just relax and enjoy your Acupuncture treatment!

Chapter 5

About Our Treatments

It is well established that the heart can produce electrical energy that is reflected through other tissue to the skin of the chest where it can be measured through an EKG. Measuring this energy is a useful way to determine some normal or abnormal functions of the heart and is performed during a comprehensive medical examination. In a similar fashion, the electrical energy of the brain is reflected through the relatively dense bone of the head to the skin of the skull where it can also be measured through EEG. Similar measurements are done through Electromyelography and Brain Stem Audiometry tests.

It should not be surprising then that other organs can reflect their energy components to the skin at various locations. However, the energy that travels through connective tissue under the skin from one conventional Acupuncture point to another is a bit harder to pin down.

Experiments conducted in which a classical Acupuncture point is injected with a radioactive substance and then followed has established that this substance can be rather quickly traced from that Acupuncture point, flowing in one direction only, to the next point following the classical Meridian pathway established some three thousand years before. That the ancient Chinese could identify these points accurately and functionally connect specific points with specific organ systems is quite a feat. This is particularly true considering that they could do so long before our current concepts of blood circulation, nerve pathways, and other anatomical knowledge and without the use of X-ray, MRI, or other modern investigative tools.

As you may have experienced, an electrical charge introduced into a human body such as someone touching an electrified fence or a car battery cable or other DC electrical source can cause a significant shock. Anyone else touching that person at that time may also feel the shock.

Recently, I witnessed an interesting demonstration in which two people held on to the metal contact points in the paws of a toy teddy bear that talked when the paws were touched together. This is much like the dog toy that squeaks when the child or dog squeezes the toy. In this instance, two people held the metal contact points in the teddy bear's paws. Then nearly a hundred other people touched them and held each other's hands in a large circle. When the circle was complete the teddy bear spoke. When someone clear across the room in the circle let go of his neighbor's hand, the speaking stopped. When they again held hands, the talking teddy bear resumed speaking. All those people were part of an electrical circuit powered by a tiny battery in the teddy bear.

When a patient is tested by the computerized electrodermal screening equipment, he or she holds a moistened brass rod in one hand while the technician touches an Acupuncture point with a probe connected to the machine. This creates a circuit with a very small undetectable current running through the patient. The amount of resistance experienced at that point or the amount of current flowing (conductance) can be measured. The patient feels nothing but a little pressure. The test can be stopped at any time if it's uncomfortable, but this rarely happens.

Variations from normal can tell the acupuncture physician helpful things about that Acupoint and its associated organ system. Not only that, but a substance, even something in a glass jar, introduced into this electrical circuit may change the point reading in a helpful or harmful way.

Imagine the benefit of knowing if an anesthetic might be harmful to a patient about to undergo surgery, or if a particular implant or dental material might react badly if used by a particular patient, or if a patient who has a reaction to a needed drug could tell if another medication might be more compatible.

In addition to measuring the resistance in a point, simply touching a particular point on a given Meridian can make a previously strong muscle temporarily weak. This would indicate a problem in the Meridian's energy component and possibly in its corresponding organ system. If touching a point caused the testing muscle to remain strong and a substance to which the body reacts, (allergy or sensitivity reaction) is brought into close proximity to the patient and the previously strong muscle becomes weak that would indicate that the body does not do as well when close to that substance. Many clinicians use this muscle testing procedure to determine compatibility to a given substance. I prefer to use the computerized electrodermal screening equipment.

Effective muscle testing, or applied kinesiology, requires good technique and lots of experience. I choose to use the computerized electrodermal screening equipment from BioMeridian, the country's leading manufacturer of bioelectrical impedance measurement devices. Over three thousand medical doctors, chiropractors, physicians, Acupuncture physicians, and other health care practitioners use BioMeridian's equipment, which is registered with the U.S. Food & Drug Administration. I find the devices' color-coded reports to be reliable and easy to understand by my patients.

Vials

We use glass allergen vials in the clinic. You can bring in foods or products that we don't have, such as leaves from a town you like to visit or your pillow. It's also a good idea to put on a dab of all of your grooming products and ones that belong to your family, or bring each in a glass jar with a lid on it. We have thousands of the vials but are happy to accommodate you in any way we can.

The vials do not contain the actual substance but rather an energetic carrier of substance signatures made by two of my favorite and trusted homeopathic suppliers. If you will be visiting a place and are concerned about the trees and flowers give me two weeks' notice and we can order the vials for you at a nominal fee.

Needles

Needling technique and needles are based on information written in about 600 A.D. We now use stainless steel needles, but earlier in Acupuncture's history, bone, bronze, tin, copper, silver, and gold were used.

Needles are inserted into the skin at specific Acupoint areas. They are gently manipulated a few times during your session and are removed in a certain way. It looks very simple, but there is a lot going on in the insertion and removal of needles. When we insert the needle, we gently move in a counterclockwise or clockwise movement. We may push it down or pull it up a fraction of an inch. This is called "manipulating the needle to activate the Qi." This is all done very gently. The Acupuncture physician feels a "tug" as on a fishing line. This tells her she has arrived at her objective. This is called Deqi. You might feel a sensation or slight pressure.

At the Acupuncture school I attended, we took classes in theory and point location before we inserted one needle. Five months after we started classes, we took a test developed by the Centers for Disease Control. We could not needle ourselves before this test is taken and passed. I have inserted over two hundred thousand needles at this time.

The needles are classified as "filiform" meaning they are solid. They have a very sharp point and are flexible. They come in different lengths and gauges. We use needles from one-half to one-and-one-half inches long and gauges of twenty-seven to thirty-one in our practice. That is about the width of a hair. We use approximately twelve on each visit, but that varies with your condition.

Needling is not the way you see it portrayed in movies. The needles are inserted just under the skin after the area is cleaned off with alcohol. We always wash our hands and use an antiseptic cleaner right before we touch you.

There may be a slight prickly feeling on insertion. It can feel like a mosquito bite, but it does not last. If at any time you are uncomfortable, please let us know. This will be a very pleasant experience and most people fall asleep.

Very rarely, you may notice a small bruise after the treatment. This could indicate a problem with your body. Some prescription medicines can cause a person to bruise easily. This is one reason we ask for a list of the medicines you take. A bruise can indicate other health conditions, but most of the time, it's just a bruise. Please bring it to our attention on your next visit. You can put an ice cube with some pressure on it when you get home.

Upon completion of your treatment, the needles are placed in a biohazard waste container as with any other doctor's office. We pay a biohazard waste control company to dispose of the needles. We are inspected by the state on a yearly basis for safety and sanitary precautions.

Cupping and Gua Sha

Cupping helps regulate the flow of Qi and Blood. It draws out Wind, Cold, Heat, and Dampness in the body.

Cupping is good for pains, problems with digestive, circulatory and respiratory systems, weakness in muscles, high blood pressure, common colds, and chest congestion. It can also be used on joints to increase the activity of synovial fluid and blood.

There are written records of cupping that date back to 2500 B.C. It has been used all over the world, and some of my patients remember their moms from Italy doing it to them as children. The cups are about the size of juice glasses. We clean the skin off with alcohol and place the cup over it. We squeeze the attached suction device until it feels tight around the area but not uncomfortable. We will do three or four cups at a time. After a few minutes, we gently rock the cup and it comes off. Sometimes a reddish ring or spot will linger and this is perfectly fine. You feel nothing but a gentle pulling on your skin. This is not unpleasant but very relaxing and takes just a few minutes.

There is a pull of very low pressure during the procedure. It is caused by the functioning of blood vessels within the muscles that are activated in response to the stimulation of the blood vessels just below the skin. This movement in the muscles allows the flow of blood and feels like a gentle pulling.

Some experts believed cupping came about as a procedure to suck poison from wounds. Some of the first cups were gourds, then glass cups were introduced. Nineteenth-century doctors in Europe and the United States used cupping for a variety of illnesses. It is still popular in Asia today. In Oriental Medicine, we talk about Qi and Blood Stagnation. Now, we know our blood isn't really "stuck," but it defines a condition of pain.

After the treatment, the skin can be pink to red for a while because of the rise in skin temperature and the increase of blood flow. We can do it safely over lung areas and along the back to aid internal organs. I had an exotic dancer as a patient and she would only let us "cup" her where she knew it would be covered. She said the cupping helped [pain in her legs] and would ask for it at least once a month.

Cupping isn't for everyone; for example, I wouldn't use the procedure on people with very fine or dry skin.

In my second month of Acupuncture school, our teacher explained a popular technique called Gua Sha. To understand how it works, we must refer back to the chapter that discussed Blood. Blood is a form of Qi produced by the Spleen, transported by the Lungs and transformed by the Heart. Blood nourishes and moistens the body and flows with Qi throughout the body. And it (Blood) gets stuck and causes pain. We call that Blood Stagnation.

Gua Sha is performed by gently running a ceramic soup spoon along your back, neck, and arms. A liniment is applied first for guiding ease. We use a short stroke similar to petting a cat. The "Sha" appears along the areas we rub. This is an indication of Blood stagnation. It can be light to dark red. It will fade in a day or so. People feel immediate relief and a looseness in the area.

We can show you how to do this at home. This technique is not taught in Chinese schools; it is something your mom would do if you came down with a cold or stiff neck. It is a very pleasant feeling, but looks like a "hickey" on your body. In fact, in the 1970s, Asian children in California going to school after receiving Gua Sha would send their teachers running to report child abuse.

I was so amazed by this technique that I spent forty dollars for a thin book on Gua Sha and excitedly told my Chinese teacher. She was mystified; she said my grandmother could have told me all I needed to know about Gua Sha. She was really surprised when I told her we didn't do it here.

Moxabustion

Every day a patient asks me about burning an herb on the end of a needle. They saw it in a movie or on a talk show. This is called "moxabustion" and is popular in

China. Moxabustion is a modality that treats and prevents disease by using heat to the Acupoints. The practitioner takes a rolled-up bit of herbs and lights it on top of a needle. This creates heat and the herbal properties are drawn into the body. A book that was written sometime during the Jin dynasty (A.D. 317-420) by a famous doctor, Ge Hong, tells of ninety-nine different conditions that use moxabustion.

Artemisia vulgaris, the herb used most commonly, belongs to the chrysanthemum family. When it is burned, the heat penetrates the body through the Acupoints and Meridians. It then activates the Qi and Blood circulation and breaks up stagnation and swelling, and eliminates cold and dampness.

In the United States, we mostly use a "cigar" shaped roll of compressed artemisia vulgaris. It is lit and held a few inches from the skin, not applied directly to the skin. It can be placed over a needle. There are contraindications such as pregnancy and the thin skin elderly people have, and high fevers. Some practitioners such as I prefer to use a special lamp with a spray version of the herb. Artemisia vulgaris has a very strong odor, and people with allergies and sensitivities can't handle the smell.

Chapter 6

Your Treatment

We follow a careful planned treatment protocol derived from years of research and knowledge of biochemistry and Acupuncture. You will receive a copy of your records; this will help you to become more involved in your treatment process. Reading this entire book will help you understand what is happening when and why. Please feel free to ask any questions anytime. It may help to write down your questions and bring them with you.

You need to eat before you come in for your treatment. Blood sugar drops throughout the day, and you might feel faint with the treatment. A protein snack of cheese, meat, eggs, nuts, or a sandwich is fine with a beverage.

You do need to avoid food and drink except water for two hours after the treatment. If this is not possible, please tell us when you come in. One patient was hosting a wine and cheese party that evening, so we altered our schedule.

If you are very sensitive to something, it may be a good idea to avoid it that day if at all possible. We have safeguards in the system to protect you, but your body still has to process the treatment and that takes twenty-four hours. The AcuSET procedure has the ability to help you achieve optimal health and overcome problems you have dealt with for many years. Patients show incredible and sometimes almost unbelievable results.

You'll recall my problems detailed at the beginning of this book. Well, after nine years since my treatment, I can still eat anything, wear anything, and smell anything without any problems. I retest myself yearly and none of my sensitivities have returned. I am happy to recheck any previous patient at a reduced fee.

Planning Ahead

I have created a sequence of treatments. Despite this, I may find something on your initial evaluation that may cause me to treat an item out of sequence.

Sensitivity elimination treatments can be performed every four hours. If you are interested in receiving two treatments in one day, let the staff know. Just remember that there is still healing time needed. Complete relief of symptoms may take a couple of weeks after your last treatment.

Appointment Scheduling

You will be scheduled for at most twelve treatment visits and a retesting visit two weeks after your last treatment. We do these treatments on Monday and Friday. You will be here about one hour. We try very hard to stay on schedule. Testing is scheduled for Wednesdays as it requires more time than treatments. We have a waiting list practice and always accommodate emergencies. If you have an unusual circumstance, please inform us and we will do all we can to help get you in and out as quickly as possible.

Instructions for the Treatments

- DO eat before your treatment.
- DO NOT chew gum or have a breath mint during your treatment.
- DO NOT wear perfume or heavily scented products in the clinic. That includes heavily scented dryer sheets or fabric softeners.
- DO NOT go to a restaurant or food store for two hours after your treatment.

- DO NOT eat or drink anything except water for two hours after your treatment.

- You may drink regular tap water except on the day you are treated for minerals. Use distilled water for two hours after your treatment.

- DO NOT kiss anyone for two hours after the treatment.

- When in doubt, check this book or ask us. If still in doubt, DO NOT go near it!

Before You Leave Your House

- Bathe and wash your hair. Use soaps that don't have strong fragrances. You may use deodorants.

- Wash your dishes and run the dishwasher and garbage disposal. Food particles can cling to dishes, dishwashers and garbage disposals. Take out the garbage.

Try not to have food on your counters or tables before you leave unless it is in plastic containers or bags.

At the Clinic

If possible, pay for your treatment when you sign in. That way, you can leave immediately after your treatment.

If you leave right away, that may lessen the chance of smelling perfume or food items for which you were treated. Sometimes people may bring in a snack, the staffers may be eating their lunches, or someone may be cleaning a room.

Toxicity and Detoxifying Treatments

People with health problems tend to be "toxic." A poor diet, overconsumption of alcohol, lack of exercise, and poor bowel habits are all negatives. Acupuncture brings the body back to health.

If you experience mild or uncomfortable symptoms during your treatments, toxicity can be an explanation. Symptoms such as mild nausea, tiredness, muscle aches, headaches, food cravings, itchiness, and anxiety are common signs. We can help with a mild homeopathic detox program. This program is inexpensive and easy to incorporate with your treatments. That can be done in a few different ways, such as a fruit and vegetable diet with some gentle herbal medicines or a homeopathic program with medicine that you would drink for a few days. None is unpleasant or dangerous. And people will feel much better, faster.

Order of Treatments

Visit 1. The first treatment is for **AMINO ACIDS**, which are the building blocks of proteins. Protein is hard for many people to digest. We believe that this is where the allergy/sensitivity problems start. We need protein to live and it is not something you can avoid. Included in amino acids vials are:

- Acid & alkaline foods
- Alanine
- Arginine
- Aspartic Acid
- Carnitine
- Citrulline
- Cysteine
- Cystine
- Glutamic Acid
- Glutamine
- Glycine
- Guanidine
- Histamine
- Histidine
- Hydroxyproline
- Isoleucine
- Leucine
- Lysine
- Methionine
- Methylguanidine
- Ornithine
- Ornithine-Aspartate
- Phenylalanine
- Proline
- Serine
- Taurine
- Thiosinamine
- Theronine
- Tryptophan
- Tyrosine
- Valine

ANIMALS

This treatment will be used if you demonstrated a reaction during the EDS testing. Most of my patients are allergic to animals. Included are:

- Cat dander/skin mix, blood, hair, saliva, and urine
- Cattle hair
- Deer
- Deer hair
- Dog (hair/skin)
- Dog hair-Poodle
- Elk hair
- Feather-canary
- Feather-duck
- Feather-goose
- Feather-mix
- Feather-parakeet
- Feather-pigeon
- Feather-turkey
- Flea shampoo
- Fur mix
- Gerbil hair
- Goat skin
- Goat hair
- Guinea pig hair
- Hamster hair
- Hog skin
- Hog hair
- Horse
- Horse skin
- Horse hair
- Mink hair
- Moose
- Mouse
- Mouse skin
- Mouse hair
- Quail
- Rabbit
- Rabbit skin
- Rabbit hair
- Rat skin
- Rat hair
- Sheep wool
- Squirrel

Visit 2. PHENOLICS are the chemicals used in thousands of products to give color and flavor, and for preservation. Some are naturally occurring ingredients. There are fourteen phenolics in milk. Tomato and soy are high in phenolics. Included are:

Acetaldehyde
Acetaldehyde
Acetylcholine Chloride
Acetylsalicylic acid-ASA
Acteylcholine chloride
ACTH
Adenine
Androsterone
Anisole
Apiol
Asparagine
BHA
BHT
Caffeic acid
Caffeine
Camphor
Cinnamic acid
Citric acid
Chlorogenic acid
Coniferyl alcohol
Coumarin
Cytosine
Dichlorobenzene
Enkephalin
Epinephrine
Eugenol
Furfural
Glutathione
Indole
Kaempferol
Kryptopyrrole
Lactic acid
Lauric acid
Lithium benzoate
Malvin
Mandelonitrile
Mannan
Menadione

Monosodium glutamate
Myristic acid
Naphthalene
Naringenin
Nicotine
Octopamine
Orotic acid
Oxalic acid
Oxytocin
P-Amino Hippuric acid
Palmitic acid
Phenol
Phloridzin
Phosphocholine
Phenyl propanolamine
Phenyl-ethanolamine
Phenylethylamine
Phenyl-isothiocyante
Phospho-ethanolamine
Pinene
Piperine
Piperonal
Potassium iodine
Primulin
Pyrrole
Salsolinol
Thiophene
Thujone
Thymine
Thymol
Tocophero
Tryptamine
Tyramine
Uric acid
Valeric acid
Vanillylamine

ENVIRONMENTALS are added to this treatment. Furniture can emit chemicals used in processing for years after it is made. Included are:

Acetate
Acrylic
Adhesive tape
Animal flea shampoo
Carbon tetrachloride
Carpet
Chlorine
Coal tar
Cotton
Dacron
Dental material
Detergents
Elastic
Fabrics
Fiberglas
Flannel
Fluorescent lights
Formaldehyde
Freon
Heavy metals
Ink
Ink-carbonless paper
Ink printers
Jute
Kapok
Lanoline
Latex
Latex gloves
Leather
Light bulbs
Lycra
Metals
Mohair
Mold
Mothballs
Newspaper
Newspaper ink
Nylon
Nylon fabric
Orlon

Orrisroot
Paint fumes
Paint-oil based
Paint-water based
Paper
Perfume
Plastics
Polyester
Porcelain
Rayon
Rubber
Silk
Sisal
Spandex
Styrofoam
Talcum powder
Tissue
Turpentine
Wood

Also on this visit, you may bring a glass jar with dabs of your makeup, toothpaste, mouthwash, and perfumes, and your spouse's and children's products. In a separate jar put your laundry soap, etc. Just don't mix things that will explode! Add some of your tap water to the jar. It won't look pretty, but we will be sure of getting your environment.

Visit 3. MINERALS are used for building and maintaining our body. We are exposed to them in daily contact. Included are:

Actinium
Aluminum
Antimony
Arsenic
Ascorbate
Barium
Beryllium
Bismuth
Boron
Bromide
Bromine
Cadmium
Calcium
Calcium ascorbate
Calcium citrate
Calcium gluconate
Cesium
Chloride
Chlorine
Chromium
Cobalt
Copper
Europium
Fluoride
Fluorine
Gadolinium
Gallium
Germanium
Gold
Holmium
Iodine
Iron
Lanthanum
Lead
Lead acetate
Lead iodide
Lithium
Maganese
Magnesium
Mercury

Mercury-ethyl
Mercury-methyl
Mercury-phenyl
Molybdenum
Neodymium
Nickel
Niobium
Osmium
Palladium
Phosphorus
Platinum
Potassium
Radium
Rubidium
Ruthenium
Samarium
Scandium
Selenium
Silver
Sodium
Strontium
Sulfur
Tellurium
Thorium
Thulium
Tin
Titanium
Tungsten
Uranium
Vanadium
Zinc
Zinc Oxide
Zirconium

✓ Drink distilled water

✓ Do not take your mineral supplement or herb for two hours.

FUELS are added to the third treatment. Included are:

Carbon monoxide
Crude oil
Diesel fuel
Exhaust emissions
Fossil fuel
Gasoline
Petroleum

✓ **DO NOT** fill your car with gas for two hours after your treatment. We don't want to expose you to the exact item for which you received treatment if at all possible.

Visit 4. EGG MIX with CHICKEN, TURKEY and DUCK. Included are:

Chicken
Duck
Egg whites
Egg yolks
Egg-fertile
Egg-goose
Egg-quail
Feathers
Tetracycline
Turkey

VITAMIN C, FRUITS, VEGETABLES, AND VINEGARS. Included are:

Alfalfa sprouts
Apple
Apricot
Artichoke
Ascorbic acid
Asparagus
Avocado
Bamboo shoots
Banana
Bean sprouts
Bean-green/string
Beetroot-beet/red beet
Bioflavoids
Black currant
Black raspberry
Blueberry
Broccoli
Brussels sprouts
Cabbage
Cantaloupe
Carambola
Carrot
Casaba melon
Catsup-tomato
Cauliflower
Celeriac celery
Celery
Chard-Swiss
Cherimoya
Cherry
Chlorophyll
Collard greens
Corn
Crab apple
Cucumber
Eggplant
Elderberry
Endive
Fig
Grape (red/green)
Grapefruit
Guava

Hesperidin
Huckleberry
Hypericin
Jicama
Kale
Kohlrabi
Kumquat
Leek
Lemon
Lettuce-iceberg
Lettuce-leaf
Lettuce-Romaine
Lingonberry
Loganberry
Loquat
Lotus root
Lychee
Mandarin orange
Mango
Mayonnaise
Mushroom
Mushroom-button
Mushroom-shiitake
Muskmelon
Mustard-condiment
Mustard-Dijon
Nectarine
Olive-green
Olive-ripe
Onion
Orange
Oxalic acid
Palm hearts
Papaya
Parsnip
Passion fruit
Peach
Pea
Pear
Pepper-green bell
Pepper-red bell
Persimmon
Pickles-dill
Pickles-sweet
Pimento
Pineapple
Plantain
Plum

Potato-red
Potato-sweet
Potato-white
Prickly pear
Prune
Pumpkin
Quercetin
Radish
Raisin
Raspberry
Rhubarb
Rock melon
Rose hips
Rutin
Salmonberry
Silver beet
Spinach
Squash-winter
Squash-yellow
Strawberry
Tangerine
Tomato
Turnip
Vinegar
Vinegar-apple cider
Vinegar-malt
Vinegar-red wine
Vitamin C-Ascorbic Acid
Vitamin K
Water chestnut
Watercress
Watermelon
Yam
Zucchini

If there is a particular fruit or vegetable not listed in the workbook with which you come in contact, please tell us. We are always happy to order new items as this can benefit all patients.

DUST and MOLD are the most common allergens. Included are:

- Alfalfa dust
- Barley-cultivated
- Broom
- Corn dust
- Corn-cultivated
- Cotton gin dust
- Cotton lint
- Cotton-aged
- Cottonseed
- Dust-house
- Elevator (grain mill) dust
- Hay dust-peanut
- Hay dust-prairie
- House dust
- House dust mites
- Kafir dust-grain sorghum
- Malt
- Oat dust
- Oat-cultivated
- Rice dust
- Rye dust
- Rye-cultivated
- Sawdust mix
- Soybean dust
- Wheat dust
- Wheat-cultivated

We have hundreds of vials of different types but you will need to bring in samples of the dust and mold from your house, car, and place of work. To treat for dust:

- Put a glass of water in each room of your house and garage for forty-eight hours before treatment. Bathroom paper cups are good for this.
- Pour a little bit from each room into one jar with a lid.

- Bring a bit of vacuum cleaner dust and dust from the air conditioning with a tissue, placing them in a plastic bag.

We each react to the different dust particles. You may not be sensitive to my dust, but could be to your own. If you forget to bring in your own dust, we can still treat you with the vials—just bring yours in on any visit.

Visit 5. FOOD ADDITIVES. Included are all color dyes, sweeteners, flavorings, baking additives, gums and starches, and:

Acacia gum
Agar
Alginic acid
Arrowroot
Arrowroot powder
Artificial sweeteners
Aspartame-Equal
Baking powder
Baking soda
BHA
BHT
Brewers yeast
Calcium sorbate
Carageenan
Chewing gum
Citric acid
Cornstarch
Cream of tartar
Dye-blue
Dye-red
Dye-yellow
Gelatin

Glycerine-animal
Glycerine-vegetable
Guar bean
Gum-acacia (Arabic)
Gum-karaya (basorum)
Gum-tragacanth
Gum-Xanthan
Gum- Xanthine
Hydrolyzed
vegetable protein
Maltol
Maple
Modified food starch
Monosodium glutamate (MSG)
Pectin
Potato starch
Saffron
Salicylic acid
Sodium fluoride
Sodium nitrite
Sorbic acid
Starch complex
Sulfites
Sulfur dioxide
Sweet gum
Tapioca
Tartrazine
Tortula yeast
Tragaconth gum
Vanilla
Whiten-all
Xylene
Saccharin
Sorbitol
Sorghum
Stevia
Sweet'n Low
Turbinado sugar
Xylitol
Yeast-baker's
Yeast-Brewer's
Yeast

TREES, PLANTS, FLOWERS, WEEDS, POLLENS, and GRASSES are treated for on this visit. Included are:

Acacia
Alder-red
Alder-white
Ash-Arizona
Ash-green
Ash-Oregon
Ash-white
Aspen-quaking
Australian silk oak
Bailey acacia
Bayberry
Beech-American
Bent grass creeping
Bermuda grass
Birch-mix
Birch-red
Birch-river
Birch-white
Bird of paradise
Bleeding heart
Blue grass
Blue grass-annual
Blue grass-Canadian
Blue grass-Kentucky
Box elder
Breath-baby's
Broom grass
Broom grass-Hungarian
Bunny ears
Calendula
Canary grass
Candytuft
Carnation
Cedar-mountain
Cedar-pinchot
Cedar-red
Century plant
Cherry-flowering
Common peony
Common zinnia
Corn pollen

Cosmos
Cottonwood
Cottonwood-Arizona
Cottonwood-eastern
Cottonwood-mix
Cottonwood-western
Crocus
Cypress-Arizona
Cypress-bald
Dahlia
Daisy
Dandelion
Dawn redwood
Daylily hybrids
Elm mix
Elm-American
Elm-cedar
Elm-Chinese
Elm-slippery
English yew
Eucalyptus
Fir-Douglas
Five grass mix
Freesia
Garden phlox
Grass
Gum-black
Gum-sweet
Hackberry
Hazelberry
Hazelnut-American
Hemlock-western
Hickory-mixed
Hickory-pignut
Hickory-shellbark
Hickory-white
Honeysuckle
Hyacinthus
Hybrids-canna
Hybrids-dahlia
Hybrids-lily
Iodine bush
Iris versicolor
Jade plant
Johnson grass
June grass-western
Juniper-one seeded

Juniper-Rocky Mountain
Lombardy poplar
Magnolia
Magnolia-saucer
Maple-hard
Marigold-American
Meadow fescue grass
Oat grass-tall
Oat-cultivated
Orchard grass
Oriental poppy
Pampas grass
Peruvian torch
Quack grass
Rose
Rosea ice plant
Rose-cottage
Rose-double delight
Rose-escapade
Rose-Granada
Rose-honor
Rose-Joseph's coat
Rose-peace
Rose-Scotch
Rose-sterling silver
Rose-yellow lady banks
Rye grass
Rye grass-Italian
Rye grass-perennial
Salt grass
Snowdrop-common
Sudan grass
Sunflower
Sweet alyssum
Sweet pea
Sweet vernal grass
Timothy grass
Tree aloe
Trumpet daffodil
Tulip-Foster
Tulips-lily flowered
Velvet grass
Wallflower
Wax begonia
Wheat grass-western
Winter aconite

✓ Do not work in the yard for the next two hours.

We have local and out-of-state varieties. If you will be traveling and are bothered by the local flora and fauna, please let us know. We will be happy to order vials for the region you plan to visit.

Visit 6. HORMONES, OILS, MEATS, DAIRY, SOY, FATS, FATTY ACIDS, and ALL FAT-SOLUBLE VITAMINS. Included are:

All Hormones
ACTH
Acid—EFA
Acid—GLA
Adrenalin
Adrenocorticotropic
Albumin-cow milk
Aldosterone
Almond oil
Alpha-linolenic acid
Androsterone
Anti Thyroid
Arachidonic acid
Avocado oil
Bacon
Beef
Bradykinin
Butter
Calcitonin
Canola oil
Casein-cow
Cheese
Cheese-American
Cheese-Camembert
Cheese-cheddar
Cheese-cottage

Cheese-cream
Cheese-feta
Cheese-goat
Cheese-mozzarella
Cheese-muenster
Cheese-parmesan
Cheese-romano
Cheese-roquefort
Cheese-swiss
Chicken
Chicken fat
Chicken liver
Cholecystokinin
Cholesterol
Chorionic Gonadotropin
Coconut oil
Cod Liver oil
Cooking oils
Corn oil
Corticosterone
Cortisol
Cottonseed oil
Cream
Crisco
Dairy
DHEA
Duck
Eicosapentaenoic acid-EPA
Epinephrine
Epogen
Estradiol
Estriol
Estrogen
Estrone
Etiocholanolone
Fat metabolism
Fatty acids
Flaxseed
Flaxseed oil
Follicle stimulating hormone-FSH
Gamma-linolenic acid-GLA
Gastrin
Gelatin
Glucagon

Goat
Gonadotropin
Goose
Grapeseed oil
Growth hormone
Ham/pork
Hydrocortisone
Insulin
Kefir
Lactogenic hormone
Lamb
Lard
Lecithin
Leukotriene
Linoleic acid
Linseed
Linseed oil
Linolenic acid
Liver-beef
Luteinzing hormone
Margarine
Meat
Melatonin
Milk-pasteurized
Milk
Milk-cow
Milk-goat
Milk-human
Milk-pasteurized
Milk-raw
Milk-rice
Milk-sheep
Milk-soya
Mutton-lamb
Neurotensin
Nut oils
Oleic acid
Olive oil
Olive oil-cold pressed
Oxytocin
Parathyroid hormone
Parathormone
Peanut oil
Pheasant
Pork
Progesterone

Prolactin
Quail
Rabbit
Rapeseed oil
Safflower oil
Secretin
Sesame oil
Soy sauce
Soybean oil
Soybeans
Sprays
Suet
Sunflower oil
Superheated
Vegetable fat
T3-Triiodothyronine
T4-Thyroxine
Teriyaki sauce
Testosterone
Thymopoetic
Thyroid peroxides
Thyroid perixodase
Thyrotropic
hormone
Thyrotropin
Thyrotropin
releasing
factor
Tofu
TSH
Turkey
Vasoactive intestinal
peptide
Vasopressin
Veal
Vegetable oils
Venison
Vitamin A-Retinol
Vitamin D2-
Calciferol
Vitamin E
Vitamin F
Vitamin A2-
Dehydroretinol
Vitamin D-
Cholecalciferol
Vitamin D3-
Cholecalciferol

Vitamin D4-(Dihydrovitamin D2)
Vitamin D-Cholecalciferol
Vitamin T-termitin
Wheat germ
Whey-cow
Yogurt-cow
Yogurt-sheep

INSECTS AND PESTICIDES. Includes all insects and all known pesticides. Included are:

American dog tick
American house spider
Anopheles mosquito
Ant-Argentine
Ant-black
Ant-fire
Ant-red
Asian tiger mosquito
Bed bug
Berlin beetle
Black blister beetle
Black widow spider
Blacklegged tick
Bloodworm
Brown recluse spider
Brown widow spider
Bumblebee
Carpenter ant
Chigger
Choriotes mite
Cockroach American/German/brownbanded/Oriental
Crab louse
Ctenocephalide
Culex
Deer fly

Demodex
Dermacenter
Dust mite
Field ant
Garden spider
Grain weevil
Harvester ant
Honeybee
Hornet
Horsefly
Housefly
Human follicle mite
Hyaluronidase
Ixodes
Killer bee
Lice
Linognathus
Mayfly
Mosquito
Mud dauber
Northern black fly
No-see-um
Notoedres
Paper wasp
Pavement ant
Phospholipase
Psoroptes
Red hair velvet ant
Red imported fire ant
Reduvid bug
Rhipicephalus
Sand fly
Sarcoptes
Scarpotic mange mite
Scorpion
Southern black fly
Southern fire ant
Stable fly
Sudan fly
Tarantula cubensis
Tropical fire ant
Tsetse fly
Wasp
Western/eastern
Wheel bug
Wolf spider
Yellow fly

Also included are flea collars and antiflea/tick medicines and pesticides and herbicides.

Visit 7. VITAMIN B COMPLEX with NEURO-TRANSMITTERS. Included are:

Acetylcholine Chloride
Amino butyric acid
Biotin-Vitamin H
Choline
Dopamine
Endorphin-alpha
Endorphin-beta
Folic acid
GABA
Histidine
Histamine
Inositol
Kryptopyrrole
L-Dopa
L-Glutamic Acid
L-Glutamine
Malvin
Nitric oxide
Norepinephrine
Orthomethyl serotonin
PABA
Phenylethylamine
Pyridoxal-5-Phosphate
Serotonin
Vitamin B13
Vitamin B15
Vitamin B17
Vitamin B1-Thiamine
Vitamin B2-Riboflavine
Vitamin B3-Niacin
Vitamin B4-Adenine
Vitamin B5-Pantothenic acid
Vitamin B6-Pyrodoxine
Vitamin B12-Cyanocobalamin

SMOKE including:

Cigar
Cigarette
Nicotine
Pipe tobacco
Smoked food flavoring
Tobacco
Wood

- ✓ **DO NOT** go near anyone who smokes for two hours.
- ✓ We will not do this treatment on a day there is a wood fire nearby.

Visit 8. SUGAR MIX includes:

Beet sugar
Brown sugar
Cane sugar
Corn sugar
Date sugar
Dextrose
Fructose
Glucose
Honey
Lactose
Maltose
Maple sugar
Molasses
Raw sugar
Rice sugar
Sorbitol
Sorghum
Sucrose
Syrup
Table sugar
Turbinado sugar
White
Xylitol

RADIATION includes:

Cell phone
Computer/keyboard
Electrical
Electromagnetic
Electrostatic electricity
EMF
EM radiation
Environmental
Etheric field
Florescent light
Gamma
Incandesce light bulb
Infrared rays
Laser
Lunar
Microwave
Monitor
Nuclear
Sun
Sun lamp
TV
Ultraviolet ray
X-ray

✓ **DO NOT** use your cell phone, computer, microwave, or TV for two hours.

Visit 9. SALT includes:

Chloride
Iodized salt
Rock salt
Salt
Sea salt
Sodium
Table

✓ Eat a good meal before you come in for your treatment.

✓ Drink distilled water for two hours.

CHEMICALS include cleaning agents and essential oils.

✓ You may be asked to bring chemicals from home or work.

✓ **DO NOT** clean anything for at least two hours.

Visit 10. CORN, GRAINS, SPICES, NUTS, LEGUMES, **and** HERBS, including:

Allspice
Almond
Almond milk
Basil
Bay
Bean-Azuki
Bean-black
Bean-fava
Bean-garbanzo
Bean-kidney
Bean-lima
Bean-mung
Bean-pinto
Bean-red kidney
Brazil nut
Caraway seed
Cardamom
Cashew
Celery seed
Chestnut
Chia seed
Chickpeas
Chili powder
Chives
Cinnamon
Clove
Coconut
Comfrey
Coriander seed
Corn
Corn blue/white/yellow
Corn oil
Corn silk
Corn syrup
Corn-red
Cornstarch
Cumin seed
Curry
Dandelion
Dill
Echinacea

Ephedra
Eucalyptus
Fennel
Fennel seed
Fenugreek
Flaxseed
Garlic
Gluten
Ginger
Hazelnut
Hop
Kamnut
Lemon grass
Lentil-brown
Lentil-green
Licorice
Macadamia nut
Mace
Marjoram
Millet
Mullein
Mustard seed
Myrrh
Nettle
Oat bran
Oats
Oregano
Paprika
Parsley
Pepper-black
Pepper-cayenne
Pepper-red
Pine nut
Pistachio
Popcorn
Poppy seed
Psyllium
Psyllium seed
Quinoa
Raspberry
Red clover
Rhubarb
Rice
Rosemary
Rye
Saffron
Sage
Sarsaparilla

Savory
Sesame
Shepherd's purse
Skullcap
Slippery elm
St. John's Wort
Sunflower
Tarragon
Thyme
Turmeric
Uva Ursi
Valerian
Vervain
Walnut
Walnut-black
Wheat
Wheat bran
Wheat germ
Wheat-organic
Wheat-white flour
Wheat-whole flour
White willow
Wild cherry
Wild rice

MEDICATIONS/VACCINATIONS commonly include:

Antiobiotics
Hormones
Pain relievers
Steroids
Vaccines

✓ Please bring in your prescription medications.

✓ If you can not take your medications before the treatment or cannot wait two hours after the treatment, please tell the staff.

Visit 11. VITAMIN A, BETA CAROTENE, FISH, AND SHELLFISH MIX. This includes:

- Abalone
- Albacore
- All forms of Vitamin A
- Anchovy
- Bass
- Bass-black
- Calamari
- Catfish
- Caviar
- Clams
- Codfish
- Conch
- Crabs
- Crappie
- Crayfish
- Escargot
- Flounder
- Grouper
- Haddock
- Halibut
- Herring
- Ling cod
- Lobster
- Mackerel
- Mahi mahi
- Monkfish
- Mussel
- Oyster
- Perch-ocean
- Pike-red snapper
- Plaice/flat fish
- Prawn/shrimp/scampi
- Salmon
- Sardines
- Scallop
- Shark
- Shellfish mix
- Shrimp
- Sole
- Squid
- Sturgeon
- Swordfish

- Trout
- Trout-rainbow
- Trout-steelhead
- Tuna fish
- Turbot
- Whale
- Whitefish

ALCOHOL includes:

- Alcohol
- Beer
- Brandy
- Cooking sprays
- Grain
- Methyl
- Port
- Rubbing alcohols
- Tequila
- Vodka
- Whiskey
- Wine-red/white
- Wood

✓ **DO NOT** consume or be near any alcohol for two hours after your treatment.

CAFFEINE MIX including:

- Caffeine
- Chocolate
- Cocoa
- Coffee
- Colas
- Decaffeinated coffee
- Decaffeinated tea
- Leather
- Peppermint
- Root beer
- Tannic acid
- Teas

- ✓ **DO NOT** wear leather shoes or belts and put your purse and/or wallet in a plastic bag.

At Home

If you were exposed to an item you were to avoid, don't panic. Your treatment may still work, but do tell us on the next visit and we will retreat. If you feel uncomfortable or have some symptoms, you may be reacting to an item not treated yet. Call us and we will get you in as soon as possible, that day if needed.

What Happens If...

Sometimes after a few treatments, you may feel that all of your symptoms are coming back. ***DO NOT*** panic or become upset. ***DO*** tell me. It could be that one of the sensitivities you were treated for did not clear and we will retest and re-treat if necessary. Some people get exposed to an item during the twenty-four-hour time period and it doesn't clear.

If a vitamin or mineral didn't clear and you ate a food with that item, it may cause a mild reaction. Again, we will retest and re-treat. Don't worry! Occasionally a combination of items can cause a symptom to return. You may be fine with tomatoes and cheese but still react to pizza. This could happen because you weren't treated for flour yet.

And sometimes as the treatments progress, you become more in tune with your body. Most of the time, people feel so much better two weeks into the treatments. Just be patient and always tell me of your concerns.

Trying a Treated Item

If you are ready to try a food item with which you had problems earlier, go slowly. The first time you expose yourself, just hold the item in your hand. Wait till the next day to smell the food item. On the third day, put a piece of the food in your mouth and then spit it out. If you are still doing fine, you can eat a small piece on the fourth day.

If it is an environmental item, proceed the same way; just don't eat it. Remember the body has to process the new messages that it's OK with the items it had previously interpreted as a "bad thing."

Anaphylactic Shock

If you had severe reactions in the past to a certain item, I will not advise you to try it—ever.

AcuSET treatments are extremely effective, and patients who have experienced catastrophic reactions in the past (like me) have had complete remissions after the treatments are finished. ***BUT*** use common sense and pay attention to your body. Any return of symptoms must be taken seriously and reported to me. Medications and inhalers are to be used until your medical doctor agrees you no longer need them.

Missed Appointments

If you can't keep your appointment, we need to know as soon as possible. We don't charge for missed appointments; I count on your consideration and respect for others. Please don't change your appointment with us because "something" came up such as a friend or relative is visiting or another appointment was changed. This is an important procedure and you need to commit to it. You can bring your friend and/or relatives and we will be happy to explain Acupuncture to them.

You may always check with me before you leave regarding your next appointment. I keep a copy of your calendar in your file. I will also know if you skip appointments. Missing appointments can slow your progress. Each treatment builds on the previous ones. If you miss three appointments, you and I will discuss your case and you may be released from care. I can't help you if you don't want to help yourself. This technique works, but you need to be here for the treatments.

Chapter 7

Testimonials

Ms. C. B. came to our clinic at the urging of her sister. She suffered with dry skin, burning feet, and itchy skin and feet; her hair was falling out and she had skin rashes. She had lived with dizziness, constipation and difficult bowel movements, headaches, pain in most of her joints, queasiness, sneezing attacks, nightmares, numbness in her hands and feet, heavy breathing, yawning in the afternoons, ankles swelling at night, shortness of breath, cramps at night, indigestion, ringing in her ears, vomiting, poor circulation, and frequent urination. She caught cold easily, gagged easily, bruised easily, couldn't relax, and felt jumpy. Lights and sounds bothered her. She was pale, and she was tired all the time.

She also told me that she had seen many, many doctors over the years with very little relief. She complained that they never listened to her or took her seriously. The medicines they prescribed caused other problems. I examined her in accordance with the Oriental Medicine Exams (pulse on all 12 Meridians, tongue diagnosis and palpitation).

We then conducted the Meridian Stress Assessment Test (MSA) and the Food and Environmental Sensitivity Assessment Test (FESA). The MSA showed Meridians that corresponded with the pulse and tongue diagnosis of her health problems. Her FESA results showed multiple sensitivities, none of which was a surprise to her.

After two AcuSET treatments, C. B. said she could see positive changes. After three weeks of treatments, she told our staff that she was delighted as many of her symptoms were going away. After a month of treatments, she was released from active care; C. B. told me that almost all of her symptoms were gone and she was going out of town for two months. It was beautiful to see the positive changes in her!

I have the privilege of seeing her occasionally in town. She moves quickly and easily, smiles a lot, and rarely has any problems with her health. She feels that for the last three and a half years, she has been living life as it should be lived.

Pain

A seventy-nine-year-old woman came to see us last year. Six physicians had treated her in the past fifteen months.

She had had twelve medical procedures and numerous prescription medicines for arm and leg pain that was so severe it interfered with her life. This also caused serious sleep problems. Her physicians ordered numerous tests, and all the results came back with no diagnosis to explain her pain. She was told there was nothing wrong with her.

As she sat in front of me, she was so bent over that she could hardly talk. There was no sparkle in her eye, and she didn't smile. Her voice was so weak that it was difficult to hear her talk. We had to help her fill out the intake form. After my usual examination including pulse (almost non-existent) and tongue diagnosis, we finally got her up on the table. I was about to tell her I didn't think I could help her but I saw the desperation in her eyes and she told me I was her last hope. I agreed to treat her for four visits and then we would determine if Acupuncture would be the right way to proceed.

After four treatments, Mrs. H. B. reported that she slept well the night before, the first time in a very long time. She had developed a sinus condition and a cough, so I treated her for that as well. I also sent her to her physician because she was in such a weakened state I was afraid she would develop something more serious. Her physician told her it was her allergies.

Mrs. H. B. had heard about the treatment we did for sensitivities and wanted to try it. I agreed and we tested her. The test results showed multiple sensitivities and we started elimination treatment that day.

I have included her actual testimonial here. I wish everyone could see this dynamo now. She travels, works part-time and is active in her neighborhood. She comes for "tune-up" treatments and at times shows up to give me a much-welcomed hug! Mrs. H. B. will always be a reminder to me that Acupuncture and AcuSET are powerful tools in helping the body repair itself, no matter how sickly or "old" a person is.

Dear Debra (Doc Rusty) Gaffney,

Thank you for restoring me, a seventy-nine-plus-year-old lady, to good health.

Before my first visit with you in February 2006, six doctors and specialists treated me for fifteen months. In that period of time, I had twelve medical procedures, blood work, and prescriptions for arm and leg pain and a serious sleep problem. All the tests were negative, and I was told there was nothing wrong with me.

On my first visit for a consultation, I could hardly walk, had no energy or strength, and could not think clearly. After three weeks of treatment, there was a big improvement in my sleep, my energy level, strength, and alertness. The arm pain was completely gone. Getting rid of the pain in my legs due to a muscle problem caused by cholesterol medicine took a little longer, but now I no longer use a cane and can once again exercise on the treadmill and other equipment.

I am now on a Maintenance Schedule and enjoying good health, something I had not experienced for many years.

Forever Grateful, H. B.

Another sweet lady, D. W., came to us with years of pain, mostly in her knees. After a few treatments, we both agreed the problem might be allergy related. We ran the test and found numerous sensitivities. She sent me a note recently saying that after her treatments she is a "very happy person. D. W." She has sent numerous people to our clinic and keeps a regular "tune-up" appointment to keep her Meridians working.

Palpitations

Mrs. A. B. had lifelong allergy problems with many food and environmental items. She was tested by conventional methods every time she changed doctors and was always told to stay away from the items that caused her problems. By the time I saw her, the years had taken a toll on her body and emotions.

Her main concern was heart palpitations, which occurred when she ate anything with red dye. She would try very hard not to eat red dye, but the medicine she had to take daily for the heart palpitations was a capsule with the company's name written in RED dye. Every morning this dear woman would scrape off as much of the name as possible with a razor.

Understanding the nature of allergies and sensitivities would explain why this was a bad idea, although clever one. Being exposed in any way causes the body to react, and this is one reason why she was not getting better.

The computerized electrodermal screening and Food and Environmental Sensitivity testing showed that she was not as sensitive as she thought to everything, but the reaction to the red dye was extreme. When we treated her for the red dye I cautioned her to do nothing but sit in a chair for twenty-five hours (the NAET way) and not to go near anything that might have any coloring in it at all. She returned in two days and we checked the red dye on the computer and the reaction was *WORSE!* We treated her again for the dyes and I sent her home with the same instructions as before. Mrs. A. B. assured me that she hadn't eaten anything with color in it or been in her kitchen for twenty-five hours. *And* she wasn't sure I knew what I was doing!

The next day, she called me and said she had reached down the side of her chair to look for something and pulled out an old candy cane. Her grandchildren had been there at Christmas. This was the very chair I had told her not to move from for twenty-five hours! The red dye had been next to her all the time.

We treated her that day with the vials and the candy cane. I wasn't taking any chances! She returned in three days and we retested her; red dye was negative! I told her not to eat anything with red dye in it. She had stopped getting palpitations.

Six years later, Mrs. A. B. came to see us for a sinus condition. I offered to retest her for the sake of my research and she agreed. All the items for which we had treated her were still negative. We found some items for which we had not treated her and proceeded to eliminate them.

Anxiety

V. R. was eighty at the time of her first visit. She wanted to try Acupuncture for her anxiety attacks. During an intense consultation, I learned she had had dangerously high blood pressure for some time. Her medications could not keep her regulated. She suffered from dizziness, anxiety, rashes, headaches, sinus problems, lack of appetite, blood sugar, joint pains, panic attacks, and insomnia.

I agreed to try to help her and we tested her on the computer. She had numerous sensitivities. During the early part of treatment, she had an emergency heart bypass operation. After she recovered from that, she returned for treatments. She felt the Acupuncture helped her recover more quickly and was eager to continue. In two months, she believed her symptoms were much improved. Afterward, she would occasionally come in for a treatment with a food item she thought was bothering her. The year before she moved away, her medical doctor told her she was in good health; she told him she credited Acupuncture!

Fibromyalgia

Ms. L. E. was plagued with severe and constant pain from fibromyalgia, chronic fevers, migraines, blurred vision, and depression. We tested her with the MSA and FESA equipment. We determined that her Meridians were in a very weakened state; specifically the Meridian pertaining to her nervous system and adrenal glands. Her most reactive food-related items were eggs, baking soda, yeast, corn, grains, salt, food colorings, and additives. Her environmental sensitivities were paper, ink, dust, and household chemicals. I asked what had happened to her before the fibromyalgia symptoms started; she remembered a very bad fall. I have observed that people with fibromyalgia and chronic fatigue often had an injury of some sort one or two years before.

L. E. hardly slept and usually could do nothing more than lie in bed. She was in the prime of her life, and this was not how she wanted to live. She had contacted numerous doctors and continued to have multiple physical symptoms.

After being treated for three months, she asked me for a letter of recommendation for a school application. Her pain, which had been overwhelming at times, now was almost completely gone. She could work for eight hours a day and still function at night. She completed her post-graduate work, kept an excellent grade average, impressed her teachers, and now is a successful and caring physician. Five years after treatment, she still was working and living a full life!

S. C. had been diagnosed with fibromyalgia five years earlier and with allergies thirteen years before that. Her job and family duties were difficult for her to complete. S. C. was taking six medications prescribed by her medical doctor with no relief from her pain. The pain level stayed at ten on a scale of one to ten.

The computerized electrodermal screening and Food and Environmental Sensitivity Assessment (FESA) results showed weakened Meridians all though the body. In fact, they were so weakened that they barely registered. S. C.'s sensitivity results were quite numerous and very high. Due to her health problems and family obligations it took six months to finish the treatments. Throughout this time, she was amazed at how well she was feeling and how strong her immune system was becoming. I talked to her six months after her last treatment, and she said she no longer had fibromyalgia!

Digestive Problems

Mrs. J. F. would experience embarrassing and distressing digestive and bowel symptoms when eating certain foods, mostly at banquets, which she attended regularly.

After identifying and eliminating the sensitivities, she was able to eat anything and enjoy her life more fully. Six years later, she still is "just fine." Here is her testimonial:

> *I cannot thank you enough for taking the time and putting me through the sensitivity procedure. For the first time in many years, I was able to attend a weekend of banquets and not worry about getting sick or just not eating. I recently spent three days in New Orleans. I ate cream sauces, steaks with a little fat, food with spices, and very rich desserts. What a wonderful time I had! With every bite, I said a prayer of thanks for you. It was such a great feeling, I am sorry I waited so long! J. F.*

A medical doctor had diagnosed A. G., a fifty-five-year-old woman, with allergies, leaky gut syndrome, insulin resistance, inflammation, and dental problems. The foods that made her symptoms worse were dairy, breads, and yeast.

A. G. was also overweight, but her family attested to the fact she did not eat much at all. She also had sleep disturbances, shortness of breath, acid reflux, bad breath, diarrhea, constipation, neck and low back pain, hair loss, and bladder problems. She did not have heart or blood pressure problems. She told me that she was "very joyful" and not emotionally affected by her health problems.

When she was tested with the computerized electrodermal screening and for food and environmental sensitivities, she reacted to foods, perfumes, trees, and paint. This did not surprise her. After six weeks of treatment, she reported feeling great and able to eat anything!

Headaches

D. C. had daily recurring headaches for seventeen years. Work, stress, and lack of sleep made them worse. She worked with children and would pick up any cold or flu that came around. When D. C. came to me, she was having headaches, stiff neck and shoulders, sore throats, low back pain, and digestive problems. She said she was always in pain, and rarely slept through a night.

After computerized electrodermal screening, we determined she had multiple sensitivities and her Meridians were in either a weakened or stressed excess state. We began treating her with the AcuSET procedure with quick response. Six months later, she had experienced only a couple of slight headaches, mostly associated with a flu episode. She no longer was catching every "bug" that came near her.

M. E. came to us with a medical diagnosis of allergies. Fifteen minutes after going into the store where she worked, she would get a headache across her forehead and a runny nose. Some of her coworkers also were complaining of symptoms. They were all sure the cause was the printed paper bags they used.

I agreed to treat her for the bags without going through the usual testing procedures. While we were sitting in my consultation room with the bags lying on my desk, I got a headache. The bags had a strong chemical odor that caused my eyes and throat to burn. I quickly treated her for the bags, and treated myself as well at the end of the day. I had to leave the office for twenty-five hours to avoid being exposed to them.

When I returned the next workday, I could still smell the ink but I did not get a headache. I called M. E.; she said she was no longer getting headaches at work and wanted to be treated for other items.

After completing the course of treatments, she noticed her stomach did not bloat and she could eat chocolate without problems. This treatment resulted in other coworkers coming in and many referrals of delightful patients over the years!

A gentleman came to us complaining of headaches from eating wheat. Other members of his family suffered from the same problem. He would also experience skin rashes, gas, hiccups, bad breath, diarrhea, dandruff, itching, and fungal infections. As a child, he would get earaches if he ate wheat. This man went to great lengths his entire adult life to avoid any wheat as well as products that had wheat in them. He found out there is wheat in soy sauce. After treatment, he was able to eat wheat three times a week or so without a slight reaction. (We encourage people to avoid items that could cause strong reactions, but they do have some protection in case of an accidental exposure.) All in all, he is very pleased with the results.

Cough

Mrs. A. G., a sweet eighty-four-year-old woman, came to me for help with a chronic cough and sinus problems. She had heard about our procedure through her hairdresser. We tested her and found twenty common sensitivities to food items. She received eight treatments and was no longer coughing. She then moved away to be with her children. I heard from her a year later and she was still doing well.

Sinus Conditions

M. F. was referred by a family I had treated a couple of years earlier. Her main problems were sinus congestion, pain, poor sleep, headaches, wheezing, high blood pressure, bad breath, and palpitations.

Testing showed deficiencies in the Meridians governing typical allergy symptoms. Her sensitivity results were quite high and numerous. After two months of treatment, she told us she had run over nine miles that week and had not been taking her medications. She told us she was ecstatic. Eight months later, she came in for treatment for slight sinus congestion but reported she was still healthy and pleased.

Another patient who suffered from sinus problems provided this testimonial:

> *Since I was in my late twenties I had had sinus problems that became progressively worse. I have suffered from sinus pain, stuffiness, infections, postnasal drip, etc. I also had headaches that developed into migraines. Since receiving Acupuncture treatments for my sinuses, I have experienced only mild headaches occasionally. The stuffiness has left and I have not had the hint of a sinus infection, nor have I had to be on any antibiotics for this condition. D. H.*

A father and adult son both came to see us for treatment to alleviate symptoms due to sinus congestion. The son could not cut his grass or work in his yard and the dad was exposed to a heavy mold problem at work. After AcuSET treatments, both were able to resume a normal life—in spite of the mold and grass.

Skin Rashes

C. A. broke out in a rash and was treated by her doctor with prescription medicines. She came to us after her rash didn't go away. She also complained of muscle cramps, cold hands and feet, fatigue, weight gain, sinus problems, earaches, teeth and gum problems (that had been treated with surgeries), and neck pain. She felt stressed on a daily basis. We found numerous sensitivities. After one month of treating her and eliminating the sensitivities, she reported she felt 100 percent better. She then had another scheduled surgery on her gums and was impressed at how quickly her gums healed.

A man came to see me for treatment of a soy allergy. He had seen many doctors and tried many medicines without much relief. He avoided soy products but, as I mentioned before, some people can react just being near the product.

His most severe complaint involved his skin. He had rashes on his hands. His face and tongue would swell. He came in one day during the treatment series in a severe situation. He could breathe but his face looked like it would crack at any time. The swelling was unbelievable.

I immediately started treatment and in a short time the swelling was subsiding. However, soy was not his most reactive item. He also had sensitivities to food additives, food colorings, grains, caffeine, chemicals, and more, and we treated him for all of them. It took three months for the skin rash to improve; skin takes a long time to heal. In four months, his hands looked good. He was no longer catching colds and his tongue rarely swelled up. He continues to come in three or four times a year, usually with something new and "strange" that he ate, but his reactions are not nearly as severe as they were.

If your favorite food or other product says "new and improved," beware! Any changes in processing or new ingredients may affect you.

C. R. came to see us six months after the 2004 Florida hurricanes. She said she had not had health problems before the hurricanes and was sure they were to blame for a rash that covered her entire face and neck. Her eyes were almost swollen shut. She would have trouble breathing and had a cough. She had tried everything. Over a course of two months of treatment, she was relieved of her rash and the horrible itching. Her breathing became normal and her cough was gone. We still don't know the cause, but we eliminated all her sensitivities as well and she was very pleased.

Hearing Problems

C. T. drove four hours to our clinic. She had been diagnosed with allergies that affected her hearing. She would sneeze if she bent over and had no sense of smell. She had sores on her tongue, excessive phlegm, red eyes, blurred vision, and coughed a lot. She suffered from itching skin rashes and was stressed out. She was on four regular allergy medicines, none of which offered much help.

The results from the EDS were quite high; anything we checked for had a reaction. She made the trip to our clinic for two treatments every Friday for two months. She then reported feeling much better and did not sneeze when she bent over. Her hearing problem also was gone.

Sneezing

I met the "Cat Lady" at a presentation I did for a local church. She wanted to experience Acupuncture. I questioned her and found no health problems. Then she said she couldn't be anywhere near a cat. In fact, she couldn't be near people who had cats. Within ten minutes, her eyes would water and itch, her nose would run, and she would sneeze. She had a new grandson, and the family had a cat. If she took her allergy medicine before she went to visit and they had they really, really cleaned house and locked the cat up in the basement, she could almost tolerate being there. But the medicine would wear off before it was time to take another dose and it made her feel drowsy.

She didn't know it, but I had cats. They never go into my closet and I don't pick them up when I'm dressed to go to the clinic. She started to get watery eyes while we were talking. I told her then that I had cats and that she had just helped confirm something I had heard about allergies.

I agreed to treat her for the cat allergy and nothing else. Two days later I called her. She had gone to a friend's house and held the cats; she played with the cats and got cat hair all over her with no reaction. We agreed it would be a good idea to come in for another treatment before seeing the new baby.

When she returned home, the "Cat Lady" said: "I was still skeptical as I entered my son's house. As soon as I sat down the cat jumped up on my lap. My first instinct was to shoo him off but I said, "Well, this will be a good test, it will be either a cure or I'll be a basket case. Honestly, it was a cure! I had a wonderful week and enjoyed holding and petting their cat—something I could never do before."

Pediatrics

About twenty-five percent of our patients are children. We dedicated a room just for them. We have toys, games, and stuffed animals for them to play with and to be treated for. They can sit at a child-sized table and color. We have had some children who come in sleeping and don't even wake up during the treatment. I use a microcurrent device that looks like a red flashlight to treat them. Here are some of their stories.

My eldest son and I were on three different medicines a month as well as allergy shots. My goal for trying Acupuncture was not to use so many medicines, stop allergy shots, and hopefully get a dog. A home with two boys just has to have a dog! Since we've been through the AcuSET treatments, we only take one medicine a month, stopped the allergy shots, and we have our dog! Before, I had to use an inhaler on a constant basis; now, I rarely use it. If I do have breathing problems, I reach for a homeopathic remedy and it usually does the trick.

Even when we are sick with a cold, we turn to Acupuncture. We know it works! My younger son is nine years old and has been practically raised on alternative treatments. I must say he is stronger and healthier than my first son. The proof is in the results. D. C.

The parents of a child with sinus and skin rashes sent this one:

My son had suffered with allergies all of his life, including sneezing and congestion that regularly became ear or sinus infections. The cycle of allergy, infection, and antibiotic was a regular part of our life. When he was fourteen, we decided to try the AcuSET with Debra Gaffney. Once my son had completed the treatments, his allergy symptoms disappeared. There was no reoccurrence except for one surprising event. He had been swimming in our spring-fed lake and once again was "filled up" with congestion and had a skin rash. We returned to the clinic with a bottle of the lake water in hand. Debra Gaffney treated our son. He is now nineteen and has not suffered any allergy reaction since. S. D.

This child's parents sent her to her grandmother's house so we could treat her.

My ten-year-old granddaughter had been diagnosed with an adrenal deficiency that restricted her growth and weight gain. She also took many medications for her allergies. I brought her from Missouri to the clinic for three weeks of intense treatments. Debra Gaffney's knowledge and caring attitude made the visits easy and enjoyable for my granddaughter.

The result was astounding—she gained two pounds and grew two inches! At my granddaughter's next visit with her pulmonary doctor in Missouri, her medications were greatly reduced to the delight of all of us! P. A. and family

One little girl wanted a kitten more than anything else but couldn't due to her asthma. After treatments, the family got a kitten. She sent this to me herself:

You have made me better. I think it's the "magic wand" (her name for the microcurrent device). I don't cough much anymore. I hardly use my inhaler or nebulizer. Please make my mom and sister better. I am doing great in gymnastics. Thank you so much! M. S. age six

I received this from a mom who took a chance.

I thought my son had a reaction to a peanut product he had eaten, and felt I was getting the runaround from his allergist. My sister suggested seeing a nutritionist, and remembered your name because your husband had treated her for back problems.

After reading all the information provided, we started our son on the series of treatments. He loved to visit your clinic. Although coming two times a week was sometimes tedious for a boisterous two-year-old, it was well worth the effort. He went from developing a rash from touching anything with milk to being able to fully tolerate it in his diet.

This has provided me with a newfound inspiration and enthusiasm for what can be accomplished in this field. It is amazing and disheartening that people suffer so many illnesses and spend so much effort covering up and treating symptoms without really ever understanding the origins.

One of the things that is so wonderful about your office is the wealth of information you provide through books and pamphlets. You also take the time to help your patients understand their problems and methods of treatments. You could go to dozens of doctors' offices before you found one doctor who seemed to be truly concerned and informed of each individual patient as you are. Many thanks, the M. family

It seems that most children who come to us have asthma and sinus problems.

We have treated many children for coughing. One little girl coughed once every five minutes, all day. She quit coughing after three months of treatment. Every few months or so, her mom brings her into the clinic for treatment to help keep her healthy.

A little boy who coughed all day, producing phlegm, was treated for sensitivities and quit coughing. His problems came from environmental items. We had them bring in his "blankie" and stuffed toys.

One little boy told me he wasn't mad all the time after the treatments. The guidance counselor at school begged his parents to bring him to us. He had a chronic cough, a runny nose, and very intense anger issues. He was not welcomed in school and was on the verge of being asked to leave.

One of my first patients was five when he started coming to us. He had a brother a year younger than him. Both were very sickly. They also had a younger brother and sister who were healthy. The only differences were the first two children had received all of their "baby shots." They had been fine till then.

They had been in and out of doctor's offices constantly. The mother radically changed the oldest boy's diet and he was getting better. She had heard about me and brought him in. His little digestive and respiratory systems were a mess. He had a constant runny nose and was underweight.

It took five months of treatments, but he became a healthy and vibrant child. We also helped his brother and mom get healthy.

Another boy came to us at age nine. He had had sinus problems and stomach issues since birth and was on seven medications. He had trouble sleeping and had rashes, headaches, and no energy. He was having problems with school and at home. He lived an hour away, and it took three months to complete the treatments. When we were done, he was sleeping well and had no headaches or sinus problems. His mom was encouraging the doctor to cut his medicines out because of the great improvements.

Another patient encouraged her child's teacher to bring her family to us. They all had allergies, stomach problems, elimination problems and skin rashes. Most kids in this situation also have irritability or anxiety problems. Understanding Oriental Medicine helps them to see the correlation. These children seem to be sensitive to most of their daily diet and are limited in what they will eat. It always amazes me that the items to which they are most sensitive are foods that they either eat daily or will not eat at all. We treated the whole family at once and had a great time doing it. Children are not afraid of coming here and can tell us when they feel better.

One thirteen-year-old boy had asthma and unexplainable fears. He also wet the bed. He was teased at school and was doing poorly in class. His diet was mostly junk food and he played computer games all the time. He got no exercise at all. After testing him with the MSA and FESA we identified his sensitivities and treated him. At the end of the six weeks his symptoms were gone and he felt like a new "kid."

We can help eliminate sensitivities and try to educate the parents and the child, but if they don't want to change their lifestyles, it is very hard to stay healthy. Being healthy is work, but it should be our number one job. We only get one body and it needs to last about one hundred years. Society and medicine can keep us alive longer, but at a price. Do you want to be active and healthy up to the day you die or be on lots of medicine and spend your days going from doctor to doctor?

Environmental things besides trees and pollens can affect us. The radiation surrounding us is a whole other book! People walking around with phones plugged in the ear and hooked on their waistbands have to be doing something negative to their bodies. Only time will tell us.

We had a teenage patient who was experiencing severe stomachaches and headaches. His medical doctor suggested that the electrical wiring in his house might be causing the problems, and the parents brought the boy to me. We treated him and in a few days his symptoms were gone. The parents also corrected the wiring problem in the house. That was five years ago and he is still fine.

We treat children with all kinds of problems. We've had babies in here with skin rashes covering most of their bodies. No one can touch them except their moms. Skin rashes are the hardest problems to fix, but we can do it with time.

We also have had babies in the clinic with colic, and treated them with great success.

We have treated children with autism with good results. One seven-month-old baby rolled over and smiled at her dad. Before they came to us, he was sure nothing could help her. She was so active after five treatments that we had to really watch her! That was one of our greatest days in our practice! They had to move away and I only hope they continued care for her.

We have treated children with irritable bowel syndrome and Crohn's disease. One twelve-year-old would have to use the bathroom two to three times before we could finish a treatment. Can you imagine what school must have been like for him? When we finished the series, he was so pleased!! He didn't have to run to the bathroom at all! I will never forget his face and the excitement in his voice when he told me how well he was doing!

Another teenager had large amounts of blood in his stool in the commode. He had missed a lot of school over the years but managed to keep a high grade average. After the treatments, the only food that caused problems was grilled onions.

Chapter 8

More Information

Every second, we are renewing our body. Over fifty trillion cells are constantly changing from our birth to our death. Every time we eat, breathe, sleep, move, shower, dry ourselves off, rub ourselves, take vitamins or medicines, exercise, and so on, we are affecting our cells. We can affect the process in a positive way by making better choices in what we eat and drink. We can also help our cells by exercising and not smoking or taking dangerous unnecessary drugs. If you need to take prescription medicines or the occasional over-the-counter medicines, then you need to learn how to help your body get rid of possible negative side effects.

We do have some control over our body and health or the lack of it. It is not "natural" for people to be on three or four prescription medicines at age fifty or to have a medicine chest filled with over-the-counter pills. It is not "natural" to forgo exercise due to pain or tiredness. But these are common things today.

In the past, the accepted thought by medical doctors was that "vitamin pills" were not necessary. This was true when our food was grown in healthy soil and was put on our table in a very short time. Now our foods are mass processed, fertilized with artificial nutrients, sprayed with pesticides, picked green, and then shipped to stores across the country.

If you are in that small group of people who eat five to seven servings of fruit and vegetables a day, then you are getting a sufficient amount of fiber. Getting fiber is a good thing as we need thirty grams a day for optimal health. But what about the nutrients to support our hectic, stress-filled lifestyle?

If you can't grow your own organic food or buy from a local market, then buy frozen fruits and vegetables. Frozen veggies and fruits are picked at the correct stage and processed quickly. When you cut an apple or juice carrots and they turn brown, you have just witnessed oxidation and a loss of vitamins. When you cut or tear your citrus, it loses its Vitamin C. Blanching, a quick immersion of veggies in boiling water for three minutes, kills a third to half of the Vitamin B complex and Vitamin C. If you squeeze oranges for juice, the Vitamin C dissipates in a very short time. In these cases, you should use supplements.

Grocery stores are trying to accommodate the growing demand for organic foods and can supply us with more and more variety. Be sure to let them know you appreciate their efforts, and help to educate them.

There are many more minerals and vitamins that need to be included in your daily diet than I can include here. As you read through the following pages, think about how many food items you eat on a daily basis. What symptoms do you have? If you demonstrated sensitivity to a certain vitamin or mineral, check with us before you continue taking your supplements.

Supplements

Vitamin supplements are insurance policies. In a perfect world, we would get all of our vitamins and minerals from our food, but that is not the case in our world today.

Every day, you need to replenish all the B, C, A, D, E, and K vitamins, minerals, amino acids, essential fatty acids, and cofactors. You need so many different actions going on in the body to keep healthy. If you are not producing the correct amount of enzymes for digestion, you are not receiving the vital, life-sustaining ingredients from the food or supplements. Without them, you create degenerative diseases and poor health.

Committees from across the world devised our nutritional daily requirement for nutrients. Their job was to develop a percentage of a particular vitamin or mineral that would help to prevent disease such as beriberi, rickets, and pellagra. We never hear of beriberi or pellagra in this country, but there are reports of rickets among inner-city children. Rickets is preventable by adequate Vitamin D. Drinking milk with added Vitamin D and fifteen minutes of daily sun exposure would stop this disease. Milk consumption is down across the nation and soda consumption is up. To save money and time, schools have cut back on physical education, and kids just don't go outside and play the way they used to. Therefore, some are not getting adequate sunlight.

Many people exhibit the signs of nutritional deficiencies: low energy; sleep problems, and a general sense that something is not right. Advertising tells us it is OK to have stomach, sleep, elimination, and pain problems. It's not OK! I see those symptoms marked on ninety percent of my new-patient questionnaires. People feel these problems are "normal." That's the *scary* part; we expect to feel bad and accept it, but that's *NOT* how it has to be. It is possible to wake up ready to start your day without health problems. It is possible to go through your day and get to bed, ready for another good night's sleep.

HOMEWORK: bring in your supplements and your Acupuncture physician will go over them with you. You will be able to eliminate some and possibly add others. More importantly, you will be advised on the quality of your supplements. Why waste money on inferior products? Bring in any questions regarding products you have heard about. We can help!

The amount and type of supplement you need may not be the same as your spouse or friend needs. We have different needs at different times in our life. For instance, the average woman's shoe size is eight. Look at your own shoes. Maybe you wear them down on the inside of your heels and your friend wears hers down on the outside. Maybe you put more weight on the toes than she does. Maybe you scuff yours on the heels and she doesn't. You both wear the same size, right? You both need the same amount and type of supplements, right? *NO!*

There is a guideline for the amount of vitamins you need on a daily basis. These are called recommended dietary allowances, or RDAs, and were created in the 1940s. In the 1990s, they were updated and new labeling guidelines were established. This has helped us become more aware of what we eat, but has confused most people. There are still flaws with these methods because they don't take into consideration how we overprocess food, how we cook our food and how poor our soil is for growing food. It does not take into consideration there are different needs for different people, and people are different. If we took two women who are the same age, same height, and same weight with the same jobs and marital status, you wouldn't have the same woman...just two women with similarities. They would not have the same DNA or RNA. They could have different genetic backgrounds. They could have different health histories and experiences. One may need more protein and one may need less. One may need to eat six times a day and one may do better eating eight times a day. So why would a "cookie cutter" vitamin pill be all they need?

If you are sensitive to certain vitamins or minerals or combinations or added ingredients in your products, your body will not handle them as well. One of the possible effects of your sensitivity is the body's inability to absorb and use them.

Many of my patients have found after their AcuSET treatments they were able to use less products or amounts. The idea behind supplementing vitamins and minerals is just not to avoid deficiencies, but to produce optimum health.

In the mid 1990s, a new Food Pyramid was introduced to get us to eat the right amount of foods daily. It is a great idea, but this pyramid really hasn't done the desired job. This is evident by the number of unhealthy people today vs. twenty years ago. The obesity numbers have increased as well. This pyramid recommends eating six to eleven servings of bread, rice, pasta, or cereal. A serving is one slice of bread; a serving of cereal is a very small bowl. Most people eat three servings of cereal at breakfast without knowing what a serving size is. A typical serving of pasta at your favorite restaurant is six cups, hardly a serving. Who do you know that eats five to nine servings of fruits and vegetables a day? Only eight percent of the population eats the correct amount on a daily basis. And I am not counting iceberg lettuce and applesauce!

French fries are the favorite vegetable with corn following in a close second. Does anyone really eat the squash that comes with your meals in a restaurant?

Pasta, rice, cereal, and breads are refined and over-processed. They have a shelf life of one to two years. When you eat these foods, they turn to sugar and cause insulin to increase. You want your body to manufacture the correct amount of hormones, not artificially raise them. Some experts think grains can cause inflammation in the body. Some of my patients and I have eliminated all grains for six weeks and felt better with an increase in energy. If you eat whole-grain pastas, breads, or cereals with brown rice, I would only recommend three to five servings a day.

Sugar is hidden in many foods, including salad dressings, pickle relish, ketchup, mayonnaise, peanut butter, and juices. I've even seen it listed in salt! White flour used in breads, cakes, crackers, and pasta turns into sugar. We have had kids come into the clinic screaming, running around, punching each other, and biting. I'll ask them what they ate that day and I can count on them saying they had pizza and cake at lunch. No child like this has ever said to me that he or she had chicken and broccoli that day!

All supplements are not made the same. I spend so much of my spare time researching vitamins and companies. I've bought them from TV specials, mail-order companies, catalog companies, old companies, and new companies. I have attended classes and sales pitches for everything that comes along. I have had patients give me bottles to try for my blessing because they are now selling them to all their friends and relatives. I have also thrown away supplements when I found out they did not live up to my strict expectations.

Are they expensive? No, but they are not cheap either. Being healthy is not cheap. You can buy sixty-four ounces of soda for under a dollar, and all you get is sugar that gives you a quick rush and lets you tumble down an hour later! Your favorite coffee is now two dollars a cup. If you're buying three cups of coffee a week, you could for the same amount you're spending in a month buy two bottles of a multiple vitamin and a Vitamin B complex in our clinic.

I ask my patients to bring in all of their supplements, and I can tell you who has insomnia when they do. Do you ever wonder why those products are sold during the night? Aren't you supposed to be asleep then—and wouldn't you love to sleep all night? We can help you achieve that and much more. Will you be taking "tons" of vitamins forever? No, that is not our plan. You will take some, and when you run out you will come by to get more—because you will see the difference in yourself.

Vitamin A

Vitamin A is essential for the tissues in the corneas, gastrointestinal tract lining, urinary tract, bladder, lungs, and skin. If you do not have enough Vitamin A, you can develop night blindness, eye inflammations, dry patches on the eyes, reduced resistance to infections, anorexia, crooked teeth, and poor bone and teeth formation. A common sign of Vitamin A deficiency is follicular keratosis. Keratin (insoluble sulfur containing proteins found in hair and skin) accumulates around the hair follicles and show up on the arms and legs as hard goose bumps, usually gray in color.

Good sources of Vitamin A are whole milk, yellow and orange vegetables, dark green vegetables, carrots, pumpkins, broccoli, squash, collards/mustard greens, kale, dark green lettuce, peppers, spinach, apricots, cantaloupes, and peaches.

Vitamin A is not flushed out with your urine, so some nutritionists are concerned about toxicity. However, this is rare; deficiencies are more common as you can see by the list of symptoms. It supplements the Blood and clears heat from the Blood.

B Complex

Vitamin B1 (Thiamin) is used to convert amino acids, fats, and carbohydrates to energy in our cells. A diet high in poor carbohydrates, alcohol, saturated fats, sugars, and fast foods accompanied by constant dieting and fasting will provide inadequate Vitamin B complex. No matter how we live or what we eat or don't eat, our need for Vitamin B complex never changes. Without it, we can experience fatigue, anorexia, digestive problems, weakness, muscle tenderness, enlarged heart, slow pulse rate, memory loss, confusion, inability to focus, constipation, nervous system problems (tingling, neuropathy, loss of feeling), and a reduced production of hydrochloric acid. B1 clears the Liver, dries Dampness in the Spleen and stops pain.

Alcohol can cause Vitamin B1 deficiency, and Vitamin B1 is necessary for alcohol metabolism. So, the very thing you need to process alcohol out of your body is reduced by alcohol. Good sources are pork, beef, enriched cereal, whole wheat, nuts, peas and beans (legumes), milk, spinach, avocados, and cantaloupes.

Vitamin B2 (Riboflavin)

Vitamin B2 helps cells to produce energy. It works with Vitamin B1 and the other B vitamins. They all depend on each other. Deficiencies can cause cracks around the corners of the mouth; inflamed tissues in the mouth; red eyes; tired eyes; burning, itchy eyes; and light sensitivity. It also causes digestive problems as well as malformed and retarded growth in children. Deficiencies also have an effect on our emotions, causing depression and hysteria.

Good sources are milk, cheese, yogurt, eggs, meat, dark leafy green vegetables, broccoli, avocados, brussels sprouts, tuna, and salmon. Vitamin B2 nourishes the Liver and supports the Kidney and Stomach Meridians.

Vitamin B3 (Niacin, Nicotinic Acid and Niacinamide)

Vitamin B3 has different names. Don't confuse nicotinic acid with the dangerous by-product of tobacco. Vitamin

B3 helps prevent pellagra, metabolizes proteins, sugars, fats, helps with circulation, feeds nervous system tissue, reduces the harmful cholesterol (LDL) and raises the good cholesterol (HDL).

People with low levels of Vitamin B3 could experience loss of appetite, anorexia, indigestion, bad breath, mouth sores, asthmatic breathing, sleeping problems, headaches, muscle aches and pains, memory problems, and irritability.

Good sources are proteins, organ meat, milk, eggs, chicken, legumes, peanuts, and muscle meats. Vitamin B3 soothes the Liver and Stomach, strengthens the Spleen, clears heat from the Stomach, and helps Qi to move freely.

Vitamin B5 (Pantothenic Acid)

Vitamin B5 helps cells release energy from proteins, fats, and carbohydrates. It also helps the body utilize other vitamins and increases our resistance to all types of stress by supporting our adrenal glands in the production of cortisone. Vitamin B5 clears Heat, clears the Liver, harmonizes the Stomach, and supplements the Spleen. It helps with fighting infections and with growth. It also utilizes Vitamin D to help our body make glycogen and fatty acids (important fuels our body needs). Vitamin B5 also helps us make estrogen and testosterone.

Neurotransmitter chemicals move information in our brain to our nerves, so if you become deficient in Vitamin B5, you will become tired, feel depressed, experience numbness and tingling in your hands and feet, and develop skin rashes as well as digestive and heart problems. An unusual sign of deficiency is prematurely gray hair.

Good sources are liver and other organ meats, fish, chicken, eggs, cheese, whole-grain cereals and breads, avocados, cauliflower, green peas, dried beans, nuts, dates, and sweet potatoes.

Vitamin B6 (Pyridoxine)

Vitamin B6 is needed in protein metabolism and helps in the making of amino acids (the building blocks of protein). It is used to convert glycogen (muscle energy supply) to glucose, which helps our brains function. It is a natural diuretic and reduces muscle spasms, stiffness in hands, and nausea. Vitamin B6 is important for normal function and growth of red blood cells. People on high-protein diets need to supplement with B6. If you experience carpal tunnel pain, joint pains, burning or tingling in your hands and legs, or sensitivity to light and noise you could be deficient in Vitamin B6. An unusual symptom is not remembering your dreams.

Good sources are meat, chicken, fish, egg yolks, soybeans, legumes, peanuts, walnuts, bananas, avocados, cabbage, cauliflower, potatoes, prunes, and whole-grain cereals and breads. It clears Heat from the Stomach and Damp Heat from the Gall Bladder and harmonizes the Liver and Stomach.

Folic Acid

Folic acid is one of the most common deficiencies in America today. Most of it is lost in cooking and food storage. Many medicines interfere with the absorption and metabolism of folic acid. If you experience any of the following symptoms you too could be deficient: headaches, memory loss, weakness, diarrhea, digestive problems, weight loss, irritability, sore tongue, and palpitations. During pregnancy, a certain type of anemia can develop. Birth control pills also reduce absorptions. This is such a serious problem that the food industry is adding folic acid to orange juice.

Good sources are dark green veggies (folic=foliage), organ meats, kidney beans, asparagus, broccoli, beets, cabbage, cauliflower, orange juice, cantaloupe, green peas, legumes, sweet potatoes, wheat germ, and whole-grain cereals and breads. It nourishes the Blood and harmonizes the Liver.

Vitamin B12 (Cobalamin)

Vitamin B12 works with amino acids during protein formation and is very important for carbohydrate, protein, and fat metabolism. It works with the brain, nerve tissue, and nerve transmission and is required for red blood cell production. This is the most frequently deficient vitamin in the country. You may have heard of people who needed Vitamin B12 injections.

Severe deficiency of Vitamin B12 causes pernicious anemia. Other symptoms can be loss of appetite, tiredness, dizziness, numbness and tingling, confusion and irritability, poor memory, and hallucinations. Our needs increase if we are pregnant, are over sixty-five, or have hyperthyroidism. An enzyme deficiency can cause digestion problems, and this can create havoc with your production of Vitamin B12. A severe deficiency can cause degeneration of the spinal cord and nerves as well as brain damage. It is depleted by hypothyroidism and lactose allergies. It supplements the Qi and Blood.

Vitamin B12 is different from other B vitamins in that it is not found in plants. It is produced by bacteria in the digestive tract of animals and humans or by microbial fermentation of foods.

Good sources are organ meats, clams, oysters, salmon, sardines, egg yolks, and nonfat dry milk. We also get it from fermented soybeans.

An interesting fact—Vitamin B12 is lost when we grill meat.

Biotin

Biotin works with the metabolism of proteins, fats, and carbohydrates. It helps folic acid to do its job better. Biotin produces healthy hair. Deficiencies can result in skin rashes, anemia, anorexia, nausea, and muscle pain.

Good sources are liver, organ meats, molasses, and milk. It nourishes the Blood and supplements the Heart.

Vitamin C

Everyone knows oranges contain Vitamin C. But most people don't know that Vitamin C is lost a short time after the orange is cut. Light, heat, and chemicals also destroy Vitamin C.

Vitamin C helps us make collagen, an important protein that binds muscle cells together. It is found in bones, teeth, skin, and scar tissue. Vitamin C helps prevent bruising and works with cholesterol metabolism and aids folic acid and iron. Since Vitamin C is destroyed by heat, light, and air, we usually need to supplement with capsules. Vitamin C is considered an antioxidant. This slows down the aging process in our body.

If you are deficient in Vitamin C, you may experience anemia, bleeding gums, loose teeth, sores in your mouth, joint pain and tenderness, slow wound healing, frequent colds, and/or allergy symptoms.

Good sources are citrus, tomatoes, green peppers, parsley, dark green leafy vegetables, broccoli, cauliflower, strawberries, cabbage, potatoes, and green peas. It clears Heat and resolves Toxins.

Vitamin D (D3)

Vitamin D helps with calcium absorption from the intestines and re-absorption from the bones. Vitamin D also works with the body's excretion of calcium and moves calcium and phosphorous to the bones and teeth. It acts as both a vitamin and a hormone. It is produced in human skin and is activated by the sun's ultraviolet rays. Vitamin D deficiencies produce rickets in children and osteomalacia in adults. Five years ago, we heard very little about Vitamin D; now, it is considered a "miracle vitamin." This is a perfect example of how little we know about the "world" of nutrients and their importance in creating and maintaining health.

Celiac disease (ingestion of gluten found in grains that is not digested correctly and causes chronic malabsorption syndrome, diarrhea, cramping, fatigue, and weight loss) is affected by Vitamin D because the absorption depends on bile secretion and fat absorption.

Good sources are cod liver oil, fish oils, the edible portion of oily skin on salmon, herring, and sardines. It is also found in fortified milk and cheese. The RDA for Vitamin D has been increased in the last few years.

It is almost impossible for vegetarians to get adequate amounts of Vitamin D by diet alone. Thirty minutes of sunlight a day is very helpful. Sunscreen, smog, clothing, fog, and pollution interfere with the absorption of the sun's helpful rays. It supplements the Kidneys, invigorates the Yang, strengthens the sinews and bones, and brightens the eyes.

Vitamin E (Alpha, Beta, Gamma, Tocopherol)

Vitamin E protects the lungs against oxidative damage from air pollutants and protects skin tissues, eyes, liver, breasts, and calf muscles. It works to maintain Vitamin A's integrity. Vitamin E is useful for structural and functional maintenance of cardio-, skeletal-, and smooth muscles. Vitamin E aids the red blood cells. A deficiency can cause a miscarriage or re-absorption of the embryo.

Good sources are vegetable and seed oils. Safflower oil is the best. Cooking and food processing reduce the Vitamin E content. Wheat germ is a good source, but when flour is milled it loses Vitamin E. In the bleaching process, Vitamin E is destroyed if chloride dioxide is used. Other sources are green leafy vegetables, wheat germ, egg yolks, butter, and nuts. It nourishes the Blood; supplements the Yang; and strengthens the ligaments, tendons, and bones.

Vitamin K

Vitamin K helps the liver's formulation of prothrombin, which starts blood clotting. When you are deficient in Vitamin K, you can hemorrhage or at the very least bruise more than normal. Vitamin K needs fats such as bile to be absorbed. Long-term use of blood-thinning drugs will increase the need for Vitamin K. If you are on blood thinners, you need to discuss this with the prescribing physician.

Vitamin K is found in dark green leafy vegetables.

Calcium

The average woman has approximately three pounds of calcium in her body. We have more calcium in our bones than any other mineral. It helps with bone strength, blood clotting, and electrical conduction in the nerves and heart. Calcium needs other minerals, especially magnesium, to complete the picture. Taking calcium alone will not build stronger bones. There are as many calcium supplements on the market as there are ideas on the correct sources of calcium. Calcium citrate is a great source and calcium carbonate is not.

Good sources of calcium are dark green vegetables, legumes, tuna, sardines, salmon, sesame seeds (you would need to eat tons!), milk, and yogurt. This is a good mineral to use as a supplement in combination with other minerals to support it.

Research shows that a lack of calcium among other minerals causes osteoporosis, osteopenia, eclampsia, and some forms of hypertension. It calms the Yang aspect of you, the overenergetic part.

Magnesium

Magnesium plays a role in keeping our cells working properly. It is required for the metabolism of most minerals and for the production of hydrochloric acid. It plays a major part with calcium in bone production.

Magnesium deficiency symptoms include muscle weakness, muscle pain and stiffness, spasms, tremors, irregular heartbeats, anorexia, and depression. It has been associated with hypertension, preeclampsia, diabetic disorders, leg cramps, and heart disease. Many drugs such as diuretics and antibiotics cause you to lose magnesium. On the other hand, large doses of magnesium can cause diarrhea.

Good sources are dark green leafy vegetables, nuts, and legumes. It suppresses Yang.

Iron

Almost everyone has heard that iron is needed for healthy blood and to prevent anemia. Its main job is hemoglobin formation. Iron supplements are needed for women of childbearing age and pregnancy. Some people will need supplementation after surgeries or traumatic injuries that cause blood loss. Some children also need supplementation. Iron deficiencies are discovered through routine blood tests.

Good sources are lean red meat, fish, chicken, citrus fruit, tomatoes, broccoli, pumpkin, cabbage, and chickpeas. Most cereals are enriched with iron. It clears Heat and cools the Blood.

Potassium

Potassium is the main electrolyte in our cells. There is a fine balance in our cells with potassium, sodium, and chloride. In this country, we ingest too much sodium and not enough potassium. Potassium is lost through diuretic and antibiotic use and when food is boiled. Eating foods raw or steamed in moderation is better.

Low levels of potassium affect blood pressure. If you are taking a hypertension drug that also is a diuretic, your prescribing physician will recommend potassium supplementation.

Symptoms of deficiency are diarrhea, nausea, muscle weakness, dizziness, flatulence, mood changes, and cardiac arrhythmias.

Good sources are squash, potatoes, spinach, lentils, legumes, peas, raisins, orange juice, cantaloupes, and bananas.

Proteins

Every cell in our body is basically protein in nature. Incompletely broken down proteins get into the bloodstream and can cause allergies. Almost twenty percent of our lean body mass is made from protein.

Amino acids are the building blocks of proteins and contain a usable form of nitrogen. There are twenty types of amino acids. Nine of these must be eaten as food on a daily basis as they are not produced in the bodies of mammals. These are called essential amino acids. The other, nonessential, amino acids are produced in the body.

The most complete proteins are from animal sources. Plant proteins lack one or more of the essential amino acids. If you choose to only eat vegetables and grains, you will need to learn the correct way to balance your protein intake.

Protein digestion starts with cooking the meat. This softens the connective tissue and makes it easier to chew, swallow, and break down. Next, the stomach takes over, using enzymes and stomach acid to continue the digestion process.

Whole proteins are absorbed except when we are under five months old. Infants can absorb whole proteins by their intestines, and this can create allergies later on.

Cow's milk and egg whites are two of the most common allergens. In adults, less hydrochloric acid and decreased enzyme production will cause gastric upsets.

Fats

The average diet contains more fat than necessary for optimal health. Fat is essential, and there are good fats. Unfortunately, most people do not know the difference. There is an overabundance of Omega-6 fatty acids in the average American diet. This causes inflammatory diseases such as arthritis and heart disease.

The good fatty acids can't be made in the human body and must be added daily to the diet. These Omega-3 fatty acids help the cells communicate with the genes. The good fatty acids are found in seeds, nuts, vegetable oils, nut and flaxseed oils. Essential fatty acids are also found in cold-water fish, rabbit, and wild game.

Most of the oils used today are processed polyunsaturated oils and are dangerous. These hydrogenated oils are in all processed foods. We know these as trans fats. Science has proven that these fats are contributing to degenerative diseases common today such as arthritis, diabetes, and obesity. This has created an uproar, and some states have banned the fats from popular fast-food restaurants.

Essential fatty acids are so important that the deficiency can contribute to abnormal clotting, heart attacks, hypertension, and strokes. Other conditions are arthritis, allergies, dry rough skin, psoriasis, brittle nails, hair loss, asthmatic breathing, migraines, and decreased fertility. Thirty to thirty-five percent of our daily intake needs to be fats, but they must be the correct fats.

Carbohydrates

Carbohydrates provide energy, help proteins to metabolize, and provide bulk to assist in digestion, elimination, and absorption. Carbohydrates are necessary to help us fight infections and for the growth of bones, skin, nails, and tendons. Carbohydrates provide glucose for energy for the red blood cells, brain, and central nervous system.

As with fats, there are good and bad carbohydrates. Good ones are found in vegetables, grains, fruits, and legumes. When most people think of carbohydrates, they think of sugar. Sugar is divided into two types—simple and complex. Simple sugars are junk foods—soda, candy, cakes, cookies, syrups, and white sugar. Fruits and vegetables contain complex sugar.

Complex carbohydrates are also found in legumes, peas, nuts, rice, and whole-grain pasta and cereals.

Fiber

In our Western society we have more constipation, hemorrhoids, anal fissures, diverticulosis, diverticulitis, gall bladder disease, hiatus hernia, gas/flatulence, obesity, high cholesterol levels, coronary disease, polyps, colon and rectal cancer, and varicose veins than we did forty years ago. In countries with diets high in fiber, these diseases and symptoms are rare.

If you just added legumes, vegetables, fruit, whole grains, flaxseed, and brown rice to your diet, you could change your health dramatically. The average fiber intake is thirteen to seventeen grams a day. It needs to be increased to twenty-five to forty grams a day.

Enzymes

Almost all enzymes are proteins and are produced in the mouth, stomach, small intestine, and pancreas. Enzymes break down proteins (protease), fats (lipase), carbohydrates (amylase), and milk (lactase). To promote digestion of food into particles for absorption, we also ingest enzymes from our food. There are over three thousand enzymes, and they aid in almost every action in the body. As we age, we produce fewer enzymes.

Enzymatic production can be affected by not eating enough raw fruits and vegetables, medications, illness, and traumas. Supplementing your diet with enzymes can produce amazing results in less than two weeks.

Oriental Nutrition

During the Tang dynasty (618-907 AD), the Chinese doctor Sun Si-miao said that regulating a sick person's diet and lifestyle could fix most situations. If it didn't, then it was time to see the doctor for Acupuncture and herbal medicine.

The Five Energies of Food

Another important aspect of nutrition is called "The Five Energies of Food." My favorite books on the subject are *The Chinese System of Food Cures* and *Chinese Natural Cures* by Henry C. Lu. Did you ever wonder why some people drank hot tea and felt better and some drank it and didn't feel better? It's because the energy of foods and beverages can create a different sensation in the body.

The five energies of food are cold, cool, neutral, warm, and hot. This does not mean the temperature of the food but rather the energetic temperature.

We all understand that ice is cold and hot water is hot. This is only a temporary condition. After you drink ice water, it warms up in your stomach; after you drink a piping hot cup of coffee, it cools down to about 102 degrees in your stomach. It is what happens after it's in your stomach that makes the real difference. The stomach's job is to receive food and liquid and to cook them (the term is "rotten and ripen"). The stomach is the "pot on a fire." The Spleen Meridian takes the "pure stuff" and helps create the Qi for other Meridians and organs. If you eat raw or cold foods (cold in temperature), it's harder for the stomach to cook them. When someone is sick, we tend to feed them soups. In winter, we tend to eat more soups and stews. These foods are easier to digest, using less Qi for the process.

Asians don't drink as many iced or cold drinks as we do in the United States. Starting a meal with a cold drink sets us up for digestive problems. It would be better to drink a warm drink as this would start to make a soup in your stomach.

Juices are another type of "not the best thing to drink" category. A hundred years ago, people ate an apple or two a day. They did not juice eight apples for one glass of juice. We did not have refrigerated trucks to transport juice all over the country. People in Florida did not have access to the amount of apples they do today and those in Ohio did not have an abundance of oranges. People ate the foods that grew in their area. Their bodies adapted to what was around them. Raw fruits tend to be dampening and can cause phlegm.

If you have a type of arthritis that causes your joints to feel hot, you are restless and perhaps irritable. You have intense stabbing pain. In that case, you would want to eat foods that are cooler to neutral in energy. If you have skin rashes that get worse with heat you would want to eat cool foods to lessen your heat. On the other hand, if you had been caught in rain in January and felt cold, you would do better if you had a cup of hot coffee or ginger tea. Why not a cup of hot tea? Tea is cold in nature. Ginger and coffee have a warm energy.

To know what foods are correct, you need to know if you have a hot or cold constitution. Your Acupuncture physician has already determined that with your initial diagnosis. A hangover in most cases can be treated with cold foods. People with weight problems tend to be on the cool to cold side. Remember, we are dealing with your Meridian health; do not confuse this with hot flashes or sweating.

Here is a list of energetic properties and common foods in which they are found.

COLD: bananas, bamboo shoots, clams, crabs, dandelion leaf, grapefruit, hops, kelp, lemon/limes, mangoes, mung bean sprouts, persimmon, rhubarb, salt, star fruit (carambola), seaweed, sugar cane, tomatoes, water chestnuts, watermelon, wheat germ, and yogurt.

COOL: amaranth, apple, artichoke, avocado, barley, bean curd (tofu), beer, black currants, blueberries, buckwheat, cauliflower, celery, chamomile tea, chrysanthemum tea, chicory, chicken egg whites, cranberries, cucumber, daikon (radish), duck eggs, eggplants, kelp, kiwi, lemon balm tea, lettuce, mandarin oranges, mangoes, marjoram (spice), millet, mint, mung beans, mushrooms (button), oranges, pears, peppermint, rabbit, radish, raspberry tea, sesame oil, soy sauce, spinach, strawberry, swiss chard, tangerine, tea (black), wheat and wheat bran, and wild rice.

NEUTRAL: adzuki beans, alfalfa sprouts, almonds, apricots, beef, beets, black sesame seeds, broad beans, chickpeas, Chinese cabbage, carrot, chicken egg yolk, corn, duck, fig, flax, goose, grapes, hazelnuts, herring, honey, lentils, licorice, liver (beef), kidney beans, (cow's) milk, (human) milk, olives, oysters, papaya, peas, peanuts, pineapple, pistachios, pomegranate, plum, pork, potato, pumpkin and seeds, quail, raspberry, rice, saffron, salmon, sardines, sesame seeds, shark, string beans, sunflower seeds, sweet potatoes, turnips, whitefish, white sugar, yams, and yellow and black soybeans.

WARM: anchovy, anise seeds, basil, bay, blackberries, black beans, butter, capers, cardamom, caraway, cherries, chestnuts, chicken, chives, cinnamon, coffee, cloves, coconut, dates, dill, fennel, garlic, ginger, ginseng, green onion leaf, green onions, guava, (fresh) ham, jasmine tea, kale, leeks, liver (chicken or pork), lobster, milk (goat), molasses, mussel, mustard leaf, nutmeg, oats, oregano, parsley, parsnips, peaches, quinoa, raspberries, rosemary, rye, sage, shrimp, spearmint, spelt, squash, sweet basil, sweet potato, turkey, thyme, turmeric, vinegar, walnut, watercress, and wine. Asparagus is considered slightly warm.

HOT: liquor, black pepper, cinnamon bark, cottonseed oil, horseradish, chili peppers, cayenne, lamb, trout, mustard, soybean oil, green pepper, red pepper, white pepper, and dried ginger.

The Five Flavors of Food

Foods have five flavors: pungent, salty, sour, bitter and sweet. Some foods can have two flavors such as grapes (sweet and pungent). In chapter 2 we described the Meridians and their properties. Each Meridian has its own sound, time of day, color, body system, odor, emotion, and flavor. The Lung Meridian has the pungent flavors, Spleen has sweet, Kidney has salt, Liver has sour, and Heart has bitter. These flavors can be used to treat conditions of the body.

For example, the sweet flavor affects the Stomach and Spleen Meridians. We tend to eat a lot of sweet foods in the

United States and we tend to be overweight. The Spleen and Stomach Meridians work with digestion. In Western terms, we agree that sweet foods have more calories and therefore weight gain occurs. Sour foods can induce perspiration and are good when someone has a cold (ginger tea).

In Chinese cooking, all five flavors are used. They know that we all need a little bit of all flavors, again, balance in all things. The sauce with which we are most familiar in Chinese cooking contains five-flavor spice, which has all five flavors in it. It is very subtle and can help balance your foods.

PUNGENT: black pepper, chive, cinnamon, cottonseed, dill, fennel, garlic, green onion, green pepper, marjoram, nutmeg, peppermint, radish, red pepper, rosemary, soybean oil, spearmint, sweet basil, white pepper, and wine. Slightly pungent are asparagus and caraway.

SALTY: artichoke, barley, clams, crab, human milk, millet, oysters, pork, salt, and seaweed.

SOUR: apple, apricot, grape, grapefruit, kiwi, mandarin orange, mango, olives, peaches, pineapple, plum, raspberry, strawberry, star fruit, tangerine, tomato, and vinegar. Extremely sour fruits are lemon, pear, and sour plum.

BITTER: asparagus, celery, chocolate, coffee, hops, lettuce, vinegar and wine, ginseng, and pumpkin. Slightly bitter are kidney beans and sunflower seeds.

SWEET: apples, apricot, bamboo shoots, bananas, barley, bean curd, beef, beets, black sesame seeds, black soybeans, Chinese cabbage, clams, coconut, coffee, corn, cucumber, dates, duck, eggplant, figs, ginseng, grapes, grapefruits, guava, honey, kidney beans, kiwi, malt, mandarin oranges, mango, cow's milk and human milk, mung beans, olives, oysters, papaya, peach, peanuts, pears, persimmon, pineapple, plum, pork, pumpkin, raspberry, potato, radish, adzuki beans, rice, saffron, sesame oil, shrimp, soybean oil, spearmint, spinach, squash, star fruit, strawberry, string beans, sugar cane, sunflower seeds, sweet potato, tangerines, tomatoes, walnuts, water chestnut, watermelon, wheat, white sugar, wine, and yellow soybeans.

Chocolate is bitter, so we add sugar and oils to it to make candy. These additives are dampening and can cause problems. Cola drinks are made with herbs and spices and can help digestion. But we add sugar water and drink them cold. This overwhelms the Spleen Meridian. There are approximately seven teaspoons of sugar in a can of soda.

Corn can be good to eat as it has a neutral temperature. But because it is neutral and sweet it can also become dampening if you eat it too often. Corn is the most popular vegetable in America and is used in many processed foods. *READ LABELS!* As you read the list of foods, it is easy to see why this country is in bad shape healthwise.

On the other hand, eggs are good to eat and easy to digest. Remember how your mom gave you a soft-boiled egg to eat when you were sick?

Coffee is in the bitter, pungent, and warm categories. It takes Yin and transforms it into a type of Qi. As the Qi moves outward, you feel increased energy. It can move stuck Qi and this is good. On the other hand, if you don't make enough Qi from eating and sleeping, you can feel more of this boost from coffee. People drink coffee when they are tired and this creates a bad cycle.

Did you ever wonder why sometimes drinking coffee gives you loose stools? Coffee is warm and causes the stomach to heat up, causing loose stools. It is also a diuretic and causes us to urinate more. Urination also loses Qi. So, drinking coffee is for only the hardy, healthy person. Some people find it hard to quit drinking coffee. We advise them to mix regular coffee with decaffeinated coffee to ease their way out. Now, there are issues with decaffeinated coffee so feel free to ask us for recommendations.

Movement of Food

The essence of foods also moves in different directions in the body, according to the Asians. Qi moves up, down and sideways. Lung Qi moves one way and Stomach Qi moves another way. If Stomach Qi moves up, we vomit.

If Lung Qi moves up, we cough. If the Liver Qi moves up, we get headaches. Triple Burner Qi needs to move down to keep urine and bowels working right.

This is a hard concept to understand, but humor me and try it. Foods that move upward are good to eat in the springtime. These are beets, apricots, beef, Chinese cabbage, carrots, celery, chicken egg yolks, duck, fig, grapes, mandarin orange, kidney beans, olives, oysters, potatoes, pineapple, string beans, adzuki beans, mushrooms, rice, and yellow soybean.

Foods that move outward are good to eat in the summer and are hot in nature. This helps us perspire and cools us off. These include black pepper, cinnamon bark, dried ginger, green and red peppers, soybean oil, and white pepper.

We need to eat foods that move downward in the autumn. These foods also help with asthma, vomiting, and hiccups, which are a reverse flow of Qi. These foods also tend to be cold, cool, or warm and are sweet and sour. They include apples, bamboo shoots, banana, barley, tofu, chicken egg whites, cucumber, eggplant, grapefruit, lettuce, mung beans, peaches, persimmons, spinach, star fruit, strawberries, tangerines, water chestnuts, and wheat.

Foods that move inward and are good in the winter are clams, crabs, hops, kelp, lettuce, salt, and seaweed. These foods are bitter or salty in flavor.

Common Organ-Related Ailments

If you have problems with an organ, try to incorporate some of the foods recommended.

Lungs: carrots, cinnamon twig, coriander, duck, garlic, ginger, ginseng, grape, green onion, honey, milk, olive, peanut, pears, peppermint, persimmon, radish, sweet basil, tangerine, walnuts, water chestnut, wine.

Large Intestine: tofu, black pepper, Chinese cabbage, corn, cucumber, eggplant, figs, honey, lettuce, nutmeg, persimmon, salt, spinach, sweet basil, white pepper, yellow soybean.

Bladder: cinnamon bark and twig, fennel, watermelon.

Kidney: black sesame seeds, caraway, chestnut, chicken egg yolk, clams, dill seeds, plum, pork, string bean, tangerine, walnuts, wheat.

Liver: black sesame seed, celery, chive, clams, crab, peppermint, plum, saffron, sour plum, vinegar, wine.

Gall Bladder: chicory.

Heart: chicken egg yolk, cinnamon twig, green pepper, milk, mung bean, persimmon, red pepper, adzuki beans, saffron, watermelon, wheat, wine.

Small Intestine: adzuki beans, salt, spinach.

Spleen: barley, tofu, beef, carrot, chestnut, chicken, cinnamon bark, clove, coriander, cucumber, dates, dill seed, eggplant, figs, garlic, ginger, ginseng, grape, green pepper, honey, kiwi malt, nutmeg, peanuts, pork, red pepper, rice, squash, string bean, wheat, white sugar, yellow soybeans. *WE WANT TO PROTECT THE STOMACH/SPLEEN MERIDANS AND ORGANS AND FOOD IS AN IMPORTANT WAY TO BUILD QI.*

Stomach: barley, tofu, beef, black pepper, Chinese cabbage, celery, chestnuts, chicken, chive, clams, clove, corn, crab, cucumber, dates, green onions, ginger, kiwi, malt, milk, mung bean, olives, pears, pork, radish, rice, salt, squash, sweet basil, tangerine, vinegar, water chestnut, watermelon, wheat bran, white pepper, wine.

Ailment-Specific Foods

If you have one of these problems, try adding some of the foods below to your diet.

Alcoholism—bananas, spinach

Asthma—pumpkin

Bleeding Gums—mangos, brushing with salt

Blood Deficiency—beef, chicken eggs, spinach

Burns—apply potatoes (not on open sores); include cucumbers and barley in your diet

Canker Sores—watermelon, star fruit

"Cold" Arthritis Pain—cherries

Constipation—bananas, Chinese cabbage, honey, papaya, pears, walnuts, tomato, spinach, pork, sweet potatoes (before bed)

Coughs—honey, lemons (for mucus), mangoes, peaches, pears, strawberries, peanuts (dry cough), walnuts, star fruit, carrots, asparagus, pumpkin, radish, water chestnuts, sunflower seeds, sesame oil, black sesame seeds, duck, chicken eggs, pork, tangerine, mandarin orange, thyme (to relieve cough)

Diabetes—spinach, water chestnut, green beans, sunflower seeds, beef, chicken

Diarrhea—figs, pineapple, carrots, barley, adzuki beans, green beans, mung beans, rice, chicken, beef, chicken eggs, pork

Edema—grapes, barley, adzuki beans, kidney beans, mung beans, beef, duck, saltwater clams, seaweed

Excess Mucus—clams, pears, radishes, seaweed

Excessive Perspiration—peaches

Eyes—cucumbers, tofu, water chestnut, chicken

Headaches—green onions, radish

Hangovers—strawberries, star fruit

Hemorrhoids—bananas, spinach, saltwater clams

Hoarseness—strawberries, chicken eggs

Hypertension—bananas, celery, clams, kelp, mung bean sprouts, sesame, peanut and corn oil, persimmons, tomatoes

Impotence—walnuts, shrimp

Improve Appetite—green and red peppers, ham

Indigestion—apples, mangoes, lemons (not with ulcers), pears, pineapple, strawberries, star fruit, barley, carrots

Induce Perspiration to Break a Fever—cinnamon, coriander, green onions, rosemary

Kidney and Bladder Stones—star fruit, walnuts

Kidney Weakness—sweet potatoes

Lack of Perspiration—peppers, star fruit

Low Blood Sugar—apples

Lubricate Intestines, Ease Constipation—bananas, cow's milk, figs, peach, soybean, walnuts, watermelon

Lubricate Lungs—apple, apricots, mandarin oranges, peanuts, persimmon, strawberries

Morning Sickness—apples, rice

Night Sweats—grapes

Nosebleeds—spinach

Pain—honey, spearmint, squash

Poor Appetite—tomatoes, chicken, fresh ham

Premature Ejaculation—sweet potatoes

Promote Digestion—apple, nutmeg, papaya, pineapples, plums, radish, tomatoes

Promote Urination—asparagus, barley, Chinese cabbage, carrots, coffee, cucumbers, grapes, hops, kidney beans, lettuce, mandarin oranges, mango, mung beans, onions, pineapples, plum, star fruit, water chestnut, watermelon

Relieve Thirst—cucumber, mango, persimmon, pineapple, tomato

Relieve Diarrhea—sunflower seeds

Sore Throat Pain—figs, lemons with honey, strawberries, watermelon, cucumbers, chicken eggs

Sinus Congestion—green onions

Skin Rashes—mung beans

Soften Hardness (Cyst, Lump, Tumor)—clams, kelp, and seaweed

Stomach Weakness—sweet potato

Stomachaches—papaya, peanuts, chives

Toothaches—star fruit

Urination—corn, grapes, pears, strawberries, watermelon, barley (difficult urination), celery, eggplants, chives (blood in the urine), raspberries, water chestnuts, green beans, walnuts, carrots (frequent urination), lettuce, onions (diminished urination)

Vomiting—pineapple

Foods to Help Correct Symptoms

After your initial consultation, you will be given a diagnosis. Check below to add the appropriate foods to help resolve your problems:

Blood Stagnation causes pain. To help your body heal, eat chestnuts, chili peppers, chives, crab, mustard leaf, onions, peaches, and vinegar.

Blood Deficiency needs a tonic to build blood up. Try adzuki beans, apricots, beef, beets, chicken eggs, dandelion leaf, dark leafy greens (mustard, turnip, beets, collards, spinach), figs, grapes, kidney beans, parsley, sardines, and watercress.

Cold conditions need warming: see the above warm foods list.

Dampness shows as edema or phlegm. To resolve it, eat adzuki beans, alfalfa, anchovy, barley, broad beans, celery, clams, corn, daikon radish, garlic, green onions, green tea, horseradish, jasmine tea, lettuce, mushrooms, mustard leaf, onion, parsley, pumpkin, radish, seaweed, and turnips. **ELIMINATE** from your diet bananas, dairy, juices, pork, oranges, tomatoes, sugar, and wheat as they help to cause dampness.

Heat includes fevers, hot flashes, general feelings of heat, red face, nosebleeds, dark urine, and hot hands and feet. These conditions need cooling foods.

Phlegm or Mucus can be helped with almonds, clams, daikon radish, garlic, grapefruit, licorice, marjoram, mushroom, mustard leaf and seeds, olives, onions, pears, black pepper, peppermint, persimmons, radish, seaweed, shrimp, tea, walnut, and watercress.

Qi, the most important aspect of our bodies, must always be replenished. Eat the following as often as possible: beef, chicken, cherries, coconuts, dates, figs, grapes, fresh ham, herrings, honey, lentils, licorice, molasses, oats, potato (sweet and small red), rice, squash, tofu, and yams.

To Move the Qi (stagnation causes pain), eat carrots, radishes, and these herbs and spices—basil, caraway, cardamom, cayenne, chive, clove, coriander, dill, garlic, marjoram, and turmeric.

Yin Tonics: apples, asparagus, chicken eggs, clams, crabs, duck and duck eggs, honey, kidney beans, lemon, mango, oyster, peas, pears, pineapples, pomegranate, pork, string beans, tofu, tomatoes, watermelon, and yams.

Yang Tonics: chestnuts, lamb, lobster, pistachio nuts, raspberries, shrimp, and walnuts. These herbs and spices also help build Yang Qi—basil, chives, cinnamon bark, chives, dill, garlic, rosemary, sage, and thyme.

Herbal Medicines

I am very concerned with the herbal use in America. It is estimated that twenty-five percent of the population uses herbal medicines, mostly bought on his or her own through the mail or the local grocery/drug store. I have studied herbal medicine for the last twenty years and understand how complicated a modality it is. The herbal medicines used in this practice are from the best quality available. We only use herbals from companies that can prove the quality control is top notch.

The problem with imported herbals bought through the mail or over the Internet is very simple. We do not know what is really in the bottles. There have been instances of labels stating a fake manufacturer or listing herbs not in the bottles. I know for a fact some of the herbals can have heavy metal, drugs, or allergens in them. Counterfeit medicines in China kill thousands of people each year. It is not uncommon to purchase a product that does not have the correct herb in it. It could have a similar species or use a part of the herb that would not do what you expect it to do.

The companies we deal with keep a constant watch over all the herbals imported and warn us of any potential problems in the sales throughout America. They buy and process the correct herbs and are constantly monitored by the U. S. Food and Drug Administration.

Now, on the other hand, it is estimated that over a hundred thousand people die each year in America from complications of over-the-counter medicines and prescription drugs. There are over twenty-five drugs that can interact with grapefruit. Imagine that—a wonderful fruit made by nature and you can't eat it if you are on certain medications. Fats and proteins can affect the absorption of some medications. Medications also block the absorption of nutrients. Many drugs cannot be combined with alcohol. Garlic can cause antidiabetic medicines to increase serum insulin levels. Do you know if the medicines (over the counter or prescriptions) that you use are affected by food?

The potential of a bad drug/herb interaction is rare when dealing with a qualified practitioner. We know which herbs are safe with which medications and make a constant study of this.

I will never take you off of your prescription medicines. That is between you and your medical doctor. But as you get closer to health, you may not need a medication or will need a lower dose. Again, you need to discuss this with your medical doctor and me. If we prescribe any herbal medicines, it will be with the knowledge and educational background of many years with ongoing study and research. There are hundreds of safe and effective formulas to heal any health problem. But I must know what medicines you take and when you take them. If there are any changes during your treatment schedule, please tell us.

The most important thing to remember is to take your prescription medicines and your herbal medicines two hours apart. If you are not on prescription medicines, we have wonderful potent formulas in easy-to-digest tablets. These would be a short-term herbal prescription, not a lifelong "can't live without" product. Remember—we are trying to correct your problem and let your body do the job it was intended to do!

Homeopathic Medicines

Samuel Hahnemann (1755-1843) is the founder of homeopathy. He was a German physician, chemist, and medical translator. He wanted to find a safer, gentler, more effective type of medicine. He admired the ancient idea of "like cures like." He took the two words from the Greek language for "similar" and "suffering" to describe his new health care system.

Homeopathic medicine is made from any and every substance in nature. A lot of the medicines today have been developed from minerals and/or plants. Dr. Hahnemann found a way to reduce the harmful side effects from medicines by diluting them into microdoses.

Homeopathy is very safe and gentle for all chronic and acute problems. It is also inexpensive. It is practiced in most countries. In Europe, homeopathy is a popular discipline.

In fact, you get a choice between allopathic or homeopathic medicine when you go to your doctor or pharmacy. In the United States mostly "alternative" practitioners use it.

This was not always so. At the beginning of the twentieth century, one in every five medical doctors was a homeopath. There were over a hundred hospitals and twenty homeopathic medical schools here. It is credited for saving countless lives during a nationwide flu epidemic. After changes in medicine early in the last century, the schools gradually closed. The demise is said to be due to politics and allopathic doctors with the advent of mass production of prescription drugs. Now, there is a resurgence and interest in the United States, and schools are opening again. In 1992, the National Institutes of Health appointed a group of health professionals to evaluate the validity of all alternative therapies, including homeopathy.

In this practice, we use a homeopathic company that has been in business for over fifty years and is used worldwide.

Another popular branch of homeopathy is the Bach Flower Remedies and Rescue Remedy. A Bach Flower Remedy questionnaire will be given to you to fill out in the beginning of your treatment schedule. Bach Flowers help to ease the emotional symptoms you may be experiencing. Dr. Edward Bach (1886-1936) was a physician in England at the beginning of the last century. He was introduced to homeopathy in medical school. He noticed that certain emotional symptoms would appear with certain physical symptoms. After years of research, he developed thirty-eight different flower remedies to help his patients and also the very famous Rescue Remedy. After you complete your questionnaire, we will determine the correct flower essences to use as an adjunct to your treatment.

You will find many books on homeopathy in this book's bibliography, bookstores, and your local library. Information also is available on the Internet.

Laughter

Laughter is important. It exercises your Liver, sends oxygen to the brain, reduces stress hormone levels, relaxes muscles, and sends out the "feel good" chemicals. Laughter can lower blood pressure. Smiling uses fewer muscles than frowning! Kids laugh hundreds of times a day and some adults don't laugh once a day. Laugh—you'll feel better!

Tension Releasers

There is a wonderful Acupuncture point on your forehead between your eyebrows. It is called YinTang. You can tap it twenty times to relax.

Another point is on the inside of your arm three fingers up from your wrist in the middle. You can rub it for twenty seconds to relax.

To help with confusion or on days when you can't tell your right from your left, try this exercise. Make two fists and tap the pinkie sides together fifteen times.

Never spend more than one hour at the computer without stretching.

Don't cradle your phone on your shoulder.

Breathing Techniques

One of my favorite breathing techniques is to take a deep breath and fill my stomach with air so it pushes out. Then I hold to the count of four and slowly release the air, pulling my stomach against my backbone. You can play with this until you can do it with ease.

Work up to inhaling to a count of eight, holding for a count of eight, and releasing for a count of eight. Then try counts of sixteen or thirty-two. If you become dizzy, back down on the counts.

If you have a headache or sinus pressure, try this: Inhale deeply, push your stomach out. Hold for the count of four and exhale through your mouth. Do this fifteen times.

If you are tired, try this: Close your left nostril with your thumb and inhale through the right nostril for a count of four or eight. Move your thumb and close off the right nostril and exhale through the left nostril. Do these four or eight times.

For pain or anxiety, inhale through your nose for a count of four and exhale through your mouth for a count of four. Try to increase the count until you get to eight.

The last technique to help with stress is to inhale and hold it up to one minute. This takes practice but well worth the effort.

Exercise

In my experience, most people do not like to exercise. Not exercising is not an option for us. We are by composition made up of muscles and bones, tendons and ligaments. They need to be active and strengthened on a daily basis. It releases those "feel good chemicals."

Exercise cleans out the lymphatic system, releases toxins through your sweat, and helps reduce stress. Strong muscles and ligaments reduce injury during falls and accidents. In my opinion, people who exercise regularly seem happier and more alive. It seems to me that the people who need exercise the most are doing it the least.

As soon as you have an operation, the hospital staff has you up and moving. There is a reason for that. You lose calcium if you lie around in bed. Muscles atrophy.

There is always something you can do. The very least would be to hold a soup can in one hand and slowly raise it and then slowly let it down. Walking around your house a couple of times a day is better than nothing. If you are capable of exercising, pick something you like to do for fun. Walk around the mall if the heat is too much for you. Water aerobics is easy and safe, even for arthritics. There are exercise shows on TV, or rent or buy a tape. My favorite one is twenty years old.

Belly dancing or any type of dancing is fun and very helpful. I have a patient who manages a senior center, and she says the people who dance every week are healthier and go to the doctor less. Play with your kids. We have a major obesity problem now with children. Children spend more time in front of computers and videogames than playing outside. Walk your dog; she is probably overweight.

Just get up and do *SOMETHING*. Your health depends on it. Remember, people live to a very ripe old age now. Do you want to be sickly and on lots of medicines or do you want to be healthy and active? The choice is really yours.

The Best Diet

There is so much confusion about what to eat. As you can see, not everybody can eat everything. Unless we advise you not to eat something, you can help build health by incorporating more vegetables and fruits in your diet.

Whole grains are good (oats, buckwheat, brown rice, rye, wheat, quinoa), but on a limited basis. Chicken is good for most people; beef is better for others. This is where a qualified nutritionist (we have two on our staff) can help you decide a daily plan.

Certainly, any processed food is bad for us. If you just look around, you see almost everyone with health problems or weight issues. I have read studies that say the average American eats out four times a week. If you have the "perfect diet" the other seventeen meals you might be able to handle the processed, oversalted, and fatty foods.

Our body is a magnificent machine. Its purpose all day and night is to keep you alive and healthy.

Our bodies have the right tools to do this but sometimes things go "haywire" and there is a breakdown in health.

Acupunture, nutrition, a correct diet, exercise, breathing techniques and AcuSET will help you obtain a better level of health—no matter how poor your health is at the start of your treatments. We have done it for thousands of people—now it's your turn!

BREATHE MORE

EAT LESS

EXERCISE MORE

WORRY LESS

References

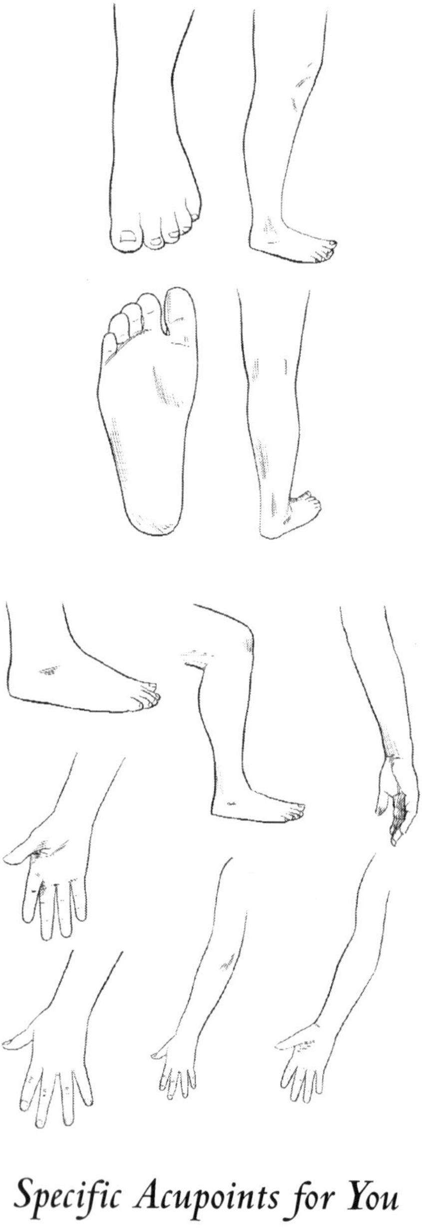

Specific Acupoints for You

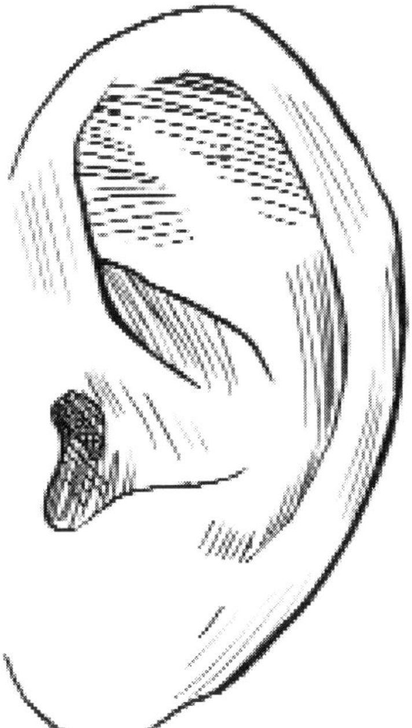

Specific Acupoints for You

Treatment Schedule

Test Date ________________ Retest Date ______________

ITEMS	DATE	CLEARED
1. Amino Acids	___________	___________
2. Animals	___________	___________
3. Phenols	___________	___________
4. Environmentals	___________	___________
5. Minerals	___________	___________
6. Fuel*	___________	___________
7. Egg/Vit. C/Veg/Fruit	___________	___________
8. Dust/Mold	___________	___________
9. Additives	___________	___________
10. Trees	___________	___________
11. Hormones/Fats	___________	___________
12. Insects/Pesticides	___________	___________

ITEMS	DATE	CLEARED
13. Vit. B Complex/ Neurotransmitters	________	________
14. Smoke	________	________
15. Sugar	________	________
16. Radiation	________	________
17. Salt	________	________
18. Chemicals	________	________
19. Corn/Grains/Nuts	________	________
20. Meds/Vaccines	________	________
21. Vit. A/Fish	________	________
22. Caffeine/Leathers*	________	________
23. Alcohol	________	________
Special Request	________	________
	________	________

**Special precautions—refer to Chapter 7*

Bibliography

Acupuncture: Everything You Ever Wanted To Know, Dr. Gary F. Fleischman, 1998, Barrytown Ltd., Barrytown, New York.

Applying Bach Flower Therapy to the Healing Profession of Homeopathy, Cornelia Richardson-Boedler, NMD, HMD, MA, MFCC, UKMHMA, 1998, B. Jain Publishers (P) Ltd., Paharganj, New Delhi, India

A Practical Dictionary of Chinese Medicine, Nigel Wiseman and Feng Ye, 1998, Paradigm Publications, Churchill Livingstone, London, England.

A Practitioner's Guide to Herb-Drug Interactions and Safety, Andrew Gaeddert, 2007, Oakland, California (study guide from Health Concerns).

Art of Palpatory Diagnosis in Oriental Medicine, Skya Gardner-Abbate, 2001,Churchill Livingstone, London, England.

Between Heaven and Earth, Harriet Beinfield, L.Ac. and Efrem Korngold, l. Ac., O.M.D. 1991, Ballentine Books, New York, New York.

Biochemical, Physiological, Molecular Aspects of Human Nutrition, Martha H. Stipanuk, 2006, Saunders, St. Louis, Missouri.

Botanical Influences on Illness, Melvyn R. Werbach M.D., Michael T. Murray N. D., 1998, Third Lane Press, Tarzana, California.

Chinese Natural Cures, Henry C. Lu, 1986, 1990, 1991, 1994, Black Dog and Leventhal Publishers, New York, New York.

Chinese Pulse Diagnosis, Leon I. Hammer M.D., 2005, Eastland Press, Seattle, Washington.

Chinese System of Food Cures, Henry C. Lu, 1986, Sterling Publishing, New York, New York.

Clinical Applications of Ayurvedic and Chinese Herbs, Kerry Bone, 2000, Phytotherapy Press, Queenland Australia.

Clinical Guide to Nutrition & Dietary Supplements in Disease Management, Jennifer Jamison, MBBCh, PhD, EdD, FACNEM, Grad Dip Human Nutrition, Professor of Diagnostic Sciences, RMIT University Victoria, Australia, 2003, Churchill Livingstone, London, England.

Cupping Therapy, Ilkay Zihni Chirali, 1999, Harcourt Brace and Company, London, England.

DeGowin's Diagnostic Examination, Richard L. DeGowin, M.D., FACP and Donald D. Brown, MD, FACP, 2000, McGraw-Hill, New York, New York.

Detoxify or Die, Sherry A. Rogers, M.D., 2002, Sand Key Company, Sarasota, Florida.

Dr. Chi's Method of Fingernail and Tongue Analysis, Tsu-Tsair Chi N.M.D., Ph.D., 2002, Chi's Enterprise.

Electromagnetic Fields, B. Blake Levitt, 1995, Hartcourt Brace, Orlando, Florida.

Fluid Physiology and Pathology in Traditional Chinese Medicine, Steven Clavey, 1995, Churchill Livingstone, London, England.

Fundamentals of Chinese Medicine, Nigel Wiseman, Andrew Ellis, and Paul Zmiewski, 1985, Paradigm Publications, Brookline, Massachusetts.

Fundamentals of Clinical Nutrition, Sarah L. Morgan and Ronald L. Weinsier, 1998, Mosby, St. Louis, Missouri.

GUA SHA, Arya Nielsen, 1995, Churchill Livingstone. New York, New York.

Heart Sense for Women, Stephen T. Sinatra, M.D., 2000, Lifeline Press, Washington, D.C.

Homeopathic Medicine at Home, Maesimund B. Panos, M.D. and Jane Heimlich, 1980, G. P. Putnam's Sons, New York, New York.

Homeopathic Self-Care, Robert Ullman, N. D. and Judith Reichenberg-Ullman, N. D. 1997, Pima Publishing, Roseville, California.

Journal of Chinese Medicine Number 9, April 1982, *History of Acupuncture*, Giovanni Maciocia.

Journal of Chinese Medicine Number 21, May 1986, *A brief study of the history and ancient literature on Acumoxibustion*, Wang Xuetai.

Journal of Chinese Medicine Number 29, January 1989, *Outline of the History of Acupuncture in Europe*, Elisabeth Hsu.

Life: Conquest of Energy, Richard M. Tullar, 1972, Holt, Rinehart and Winston, New York, New York.

Live Free from Asthma and Allergies, Dr. Ellen Cutler, D.C., 2007, Celestial Arts, Berkeley, California

Manual of Dermatology in Chinese Medicine, Shen De-Hui, Wu Xin Fen, Nissi Wang, 1995, Eastland Press, Seattle, Washington.

Micro Miracles, Dr. Ellen Cutler, D.C., 2006, Rodale Press, Emmaus, Pennsylvania.

Nutritional Support of Medical Practice, Howard A. Schneider, Carl E. Anderson, David B. Coursin, 1977, Harper & Row, Philadelphia, Pennsylvania.

Optimal Wellness, Ralph Golan, M.D., 1995, Ballantine Books, New York, New York.

Physicians Desk Reference for Herbal Medicines, 1998.

Perspectives in Nutrition, Wardlaw, Hampl, and DiSilvestro, 2004, McGraw Hill, New York, New York.

Pharmacodynamic Basis of Herbal Medicine, Manuchair Ebadi, 2000, CRC Press.

Practical Diagnosis in Traditional Chinese Medicine, Tietao Deng, 1991, Churchill Livingstone. London, England.

Principles and Practice of Phytotherapy, Simon Mills and Kerry Bone, 2000, Churchill Livingstone, London, England.

Say Good-bye to ADD and ADHD, Dr. Devi Nambudripad, 1999, Delta Publishing Company, Buena Park, California.

The Acupuncture Response, Glenn S. Rothfeld, M.D., M. Ac., and Suzanne Levert, 2001, Contemporary Books, McGraw Hill. New York, New York.

The Biology of Belief, Bruce H. Lipton, Ph.D., 2005, Mountain of Love/Elite Books, Santa Rosa, California.

The Body Electric, Robert O. Becker, M.D. and Gary Selden, 1985, William Morrow, New York, New York.

The Complete Book of Chinese Health and Healing, Daniel Reid, 1994, Shambhala Publications, Boston, Masschusetts.

The Complete Idiot's Guide to Acupuncture & Acupressure, David W. Sollars, L.Ac., 2000, Penguin Books, New York, New York.

The Foundations of Chinese Medicine, Giovanni Maciocia, 1989, Churchill Livingstone, London, England.

The Merck Manual of Diagnosis and Therapy, 1992, Merck Research Laboratories.

The New Nutrition, Dr. Michael Colgan, 1995, Apple Publishing, Rahway, New Jersey.

The Nutrition Desk Reference, Robert H. Garrison, Jr., M.A., R.Ph., and Elizabeth Somer, M. A., 1985, Keats Publishing, New Canaan, Connecticut.

The Secret of Chinese Pulse Diagnosis, Bob Flaws,1995, Blue Poppy Press, Boulder, Colorado.

The Tao of Healthy Eating, Bob Flaws, 1997, Blue Poppy Press, Boulder, Colorado.

The Web That Has No Weaver, Ted J. Kaptchuk O.M.D., 1996, Congdon & Weeds, Chicago, Illinois.

The Yellow Emperor's Classic of Internal Medicine translated, with an introductory study by Ilza Veith, 1966, First University of California Press Edition, Berkeley, California.

Understanding Acupuncture, Stephen J. Birch and Robert L. Felt, 1999, Churchill Livingstone, London, England.

Why Do I Need Whole Food Supplements?, Lorrie Medford, C.N., 2006, LDN Publishing, Tulsa, Oklahoma.

Why Do I Really Need Herbs?, Lorrie Medford, C.N., 2004, LDN Publishing, Tulsa, Oklahoma.

Winning the War against Immune Disorders & Allergies, Ellen Cutler, D.C., 1998, Delmar Publishers, Albany, New York.

www.acufinder.com/articles, 2007.

www.accpuncturetoday.com/articles, 2007.

Index

A

A, vitamin, 165–166, 174
absorption of vitamins, 170, 173
accidents, 205
acid reflux, 141
acne, 44
Acupoints, 5, 27, 73, 78–80, 82, 87
acupuncture, defined, 24, 23, 24
AcuSET
  history of, 5–15
  methods behind, 17–37
additives, food, 40, 46, 107–108, 136–138, 146, 188
adrenal deficiency, 150, 168
agitation, 33
ailment-specific foods, 192–196
alcohol, 46, 93, 126, 166–167, 192, 200
allergens, avoiding, 6–7, 12–13
allopathy, 5, 202
amino acids, 93–94, 159, 166, 169–170, 178
anal fissures, 181
anaphylactic shock, 128–129
anemia, 170–172, 176
anesthesia, 79
anger issues, 153
animals, 11, 14, 52, 95, 147–149, 151
anorexia, 165–166, 168, 172, 176
antibiotics, 54, 124, 144, 150, 176–177
antibodies, 41
antioxidants, 172
anxiety
  asthma, 53
  breathing techniques, 205
  fibromyalgia, 66–67
  as a symptom, 43, 45–46
  testimonials, 131, 137–138, 154
  toxicity, 93
appendicitis, 21

appetite, lack of, 137, 168, 171, 194–195
appointments, missed, 129
ariculotherapy, 23
artemisia vulgaris, 87
arthritis, 43, 46–50, 67, 179–180, 184, 193, 206
asthma
  fat deficiencies, 180
  foods for, 190, 192
  as a symptom, 43, 50–57
  testimonials, 151–152, 154
  vitamin deficiencies, 168
autism, 156

B

B1, vitamin, 166–167
B12, vitamin, 170–171
B2, vitamin, 167
B3, vitamin, 167–168
B5, vitamin, 168–169
B6, vitamin, 169–170
Bach, Dr. Edward, 202
Bach Flower Remedies, 202
back pain, 43, 85, 141
bacteria, 34, 41, 171
bad breath, 24, 141, 143–144, 168
balance, 24, 25, 30, 187
bathing before treatment, 92
bed wetting, 154
Ben Cao Gang Nu (Material Medica), 19
beriberi, 160
Bi Syndrome, 46
bile, 173, 175
BioMeridian, 80–81
BioSET (BioEnergetic Sensitivity and Enzyme Therapy), 9
biotin, 172
birth control, 170
bitter flavors, 187, 190
Bladder, 29, 34, 26, 65, 141, 191
Bladder Meridian, 22
bloating, 30, 39–40, 143
Blood (xue)
  defining the problem, 46, 60, 63
  methods behind AcuSET, 29, 26, 27, 31, 37
  minerals, 177
  office visits, 70–71
  treatments, 83, 85–87
  vitamins, 166, 172, 175
blood clotting, 175, 180
Blood Deficiency, 192, 197
blood pressure, 43, 84, 137, 141, 144, 177, 203
Blood Stagnation, 197
blood sugar, 11, 89, 137, 194
blurry vision, 65, 138, 147
bones, 165, 172–176, 180, 205
brain damage, 171
Brain Stem Audiometry test, 77
breast lumps, 43
breathing problems
  asthma, 50–52, 54, 56
  fat deficiencies, 180
  fibromyalgia, 65

breathing problems *(cont.)*
as a symptom, 43
testimonials, 131, 141, 146
breathing techniques, 46, 204–205
bruising, 67, 83, 131, 172, 175
burning, 131, 142, 167, 169
burns, 193

C

C, vitamin, 172–173
caffeine, 71, 96, 126, 146, 189
calcium, 173, 175–176, 205
cancer, 58, 181
canker sores, 193
carbohydrates, 168, 170, 172, 180–181
carbon dioxide, 26
carpal tunnel, 169
cats, 147–149, 151
celiac disease, 173
Centers for Disease Control, 82
Channels. *see* Meridians
chemicals
fibromyalgia, 65, 68
in food, 40
testimonials, 138, 142, 146
treatment for, 98, 121
chest congestion, 84
chest tightness, 50–52, 56
Ch'I Po, 19
children, treatment of, 14–15, 149–156
Chinese Natural Cures, 182
Chinese System of Food Cures, The, 182
chiropractic, 32
chloride, 177
chloride dioxide, 174
cholesterol, 135, 168, 172, 181
circulation, 131, 168
cleaners, 11, 93, 121
clotting, blood, 175, 180
cold, common
asthma, 50–51
cupping, 84
diarrhea, 62
Gua Sha, 86
office visits, 72
as a symptom, 43
testimonials, 131, 141, 146, 149
vitamin deficiencies, 172
Wind, condition of, 36
Cold, condition of
arthritis, 46
asthma, 50
comparison to earth, 24
cupping, 83
defined, 29
diarrhea, 60
Eight Principle Patterns, 31
foods for, 197
moxabustion, 87
office visits, 72
cold energy foods, 184–185
cold hands and feet, 65, 145
colic, 155
collagen, 172
color, skin, 17, 23, 69–70

confusion, 166, 171
congestion, 196
constipation
  Dryness, condition of, 31
  fiber, lack of, 181
  foods for, 193, 195
  Heat, condition of, 33
  irritable bowel syndrome, 60
  as a symptom, 43, 57–58
  testimonials, 131, 141, 154
  vitamin deficiencies, 166
cool energy foods, 185
corn, sensitivity to, 42
coronary disease, 181
cotton, 12, 66, 98
coughing
  arthritis, 50
  asthma, 54, 56
  Dryness, condition of, 31
  foods for, 193
  Lung Qi, 190
  as side effect of treatment, 12
  as a symptom, 43, 58–59, 143–144
  testimonials, 133, 146–147, 151–152
cracked mouth, 167
cramps, 29, 43, 61, 131, 145, 173, 176
cravings, food, 25, 41–43, 93
Crohn's disease, 156
cupping, 83–85
Cutler, Dr. Ellen, 9–10
cysts, 34, 196

D

D, vitamin, 168, 173–174
dairy
  enzymes, 181
  protein source, 179
  sensitivity to, 43
  testimonials, 141, 151
  treatment for, 96, 112–116
  vitamin D, 160
  vitamin source, 166–169, 171–172, 174–175
Damp Heat, 29
Dampness, condition of
  arthritis, 46
  comparison to earth, 24–25
  cupping, 83
  defined, 30
  diarrhea, 60
  dispersion, 31
  foods for, 197
  moxabustion, 87
  vitamin deficiencies, 166, 170
  Yin, 37
dancing, 206
dandruff, 143
deficiencies, mineral, 176, 180
deficiencies, vitamin, 165–167, 169–175
Deficiency, 25, 27, 28, 30, 31, 71, 144
dehydration, 33
dental problems, 31, 44, 141, 145, 165, 172, 196

depression, 12, 43, 65, 138, 167, 169, 176
Deqi, 30, 82
diabetes, 176, 180, 193, 200
diarrhea
  asthma, 53
  Damp Heat, 29
  foods for, 193, 196
  mineral deficiencies, 176–177
  as a symptom, 43, 45, 59–62
  testimonials, 141, 143
  vitamin deficiencies, 170, 173
diet. *see also* food sensitivities
  anxiety, 46
  changes in, 40
  diarrhea, 59
  fats, 179
  holistic medicine, 32
  ideal, 206–207
  supplements, 159
  testimonials, 151, 153–154
  toxicity, 93
  vitamin D, 174
  vitamin deficiencies, 166
digestion, promoting, 195
digestive problems
  asthma, 53
  cupping, 84
  nutritional deficiencies, 160
  as a symptom, 15, 43–45, 62–64
  testimonials, 131, 140–141, 153–154
  vitamin deficiencies, 166–167, 169–171
digestive process, 178, 181, 187–188
discharge, sticky, 30
disharmony, condition of, 30
disperse, defined, 31
distal points, defined, 31
diuretics, 169, 176–177, 189
diverticulitis, 181
diverticulosis, 181
dizziness
  fibromyalgia, 65
  mineral deficiencies, 177
  as a symptom, 7, 26–27, 43, 45
  testimonials, 131, 137
  vitamin deficiencies, 171
DNA, 162
dreams, 67, 169
drowsiness. *see* fatigue
drugs, 157
Dryness, condition of, 24, 27, 28, 31, 50, 57, 165
Du Meridian, 24, 23,
dust, sensitivity to, 11, 106–107, 138

E

E, vitamin, 174–175
earaches, 143, 145
eating and timing of treatment, 89–92, 121
eclampsia, 176
edema, 30, 193

EDS (electrodermal screening)
animals, 95
arthritis, 47
and BioSET, 9
constipation, 58
fibromyalgia, 65, 68
Food and Environmental Sensitivity Assessment (FESA), 32
Meridian Stress Assessment (MSA), 33
office visits, 75
testimonials, 136, 139, 141, 147
testing vials, 13
treatments, 79–80
EEG, 77
eggs
protein source, 179
sensitivity to, 10, 41–42
testimonials, 138
treatment for, 102
vitamin source, 167–169, 171, 174
Eight Principle Patterns, defined, 31
ejaculation, premature, 195
EKG, 77
electrical conduction, 175
electricity, 66, 120
Electromyelography, 77
emotions, seven, 35
emphysema, 58
energy
electrical, 77–81
food, 182–186
energy *(cont.)*
lack of, 14–15, 44, 133–135, 153, 160
negative correlation to grain consumption, 163
vitamin B2, 167–169
environmental factors, 30, 98–99, 135, 138, 152, 155
enzymes, 179, 181–182
essence (jing), 32
essential fatty acids, 159
estrogen, 168
Excess, 28, 30, 31, 33, 34, 71, 142
exercise
anxiety, 46
balance, importance of, 24
benefits of, 205–206
constipation, 57
holistic medicine, 32
testimonials, 135, 154, 157–158
toxicity, 93
exhaustion. *see* fatigue
external factors, 31, 34, 37
eyes, dry/red, 43, 165, 167, 194

F

fasting, 11
fatigue. *see also* sleep
breathing techniques, 204–205
control over health, 158
fibromyalgia, 65–68
office visits, 71
side effect of treatment, 11–12
as a symptom, 40, 43

fatigue (cont.)
testimonials, 131, 138, 145, 148
toxicity, 93
vitamin deficiencies, 166, 169, 171, 173
fats
absorption of medications, 200
in diet, 179–180
enzymes, 181
metabolism of, 171–173
treatment for, 112–116
vitamin B5, 168
vitamin deficiencies, 166
vitamin K, 175
fatty acids, 168, 179
fears, unexplained, 45, 154
feeling, loss of, 166
feet, swollen, 65
fertility, decreased, 180
fever, 33, 36, 87, 138, 194
fiber, 158, 181
fibromylagia, 64–68, 138–140
fish, 125–126, 167, 169, 171, 173, 175, 177
Five Energies of Food, 182–186
Five Flavors of Food, 186–189
flatulence, 177, 181
flowers. *see* plants
flu, 43, 51, 59, 141–142
focus, inability to, 166
folic acid, 170, 172
follicular keratosis, 165
Food & Drug Administration, U.S., 81, 199
food additives. *see* additives, food
Food and Environmental Sensitivity Assessment (FESA)
asthma, 53
constipation, 58
coughing, 59
defined, 32
office visits, 75
testimonials, 132, 136, 138–139, 141, 154
food coloring, 46, 138, 146
Food Pyramid, 162
food sensitivities, 39–43, 91–93, 135, 141. *see also* diet
formaldehyde, 43, 66, 98
fuels, 102
fungi, 34, 143

G

Gaffney, John, 6
gagging, 131
Gall Bladder, 29, 34, 36, 73, 170, 181, 191
Gall Bladder Meridian, 22
gallstones, 29
gas, 44, 143, 181
Ge Hong, 87
GERD, 63
glucose, 169, 180
gluten, 173
glycogen, 168–169
grains
mineral source, 177
negative correlation to energy, 163–164

grains *(cont.)*
sensitivity to, 8–11, 47
testimonials, 138, 141, 143, 146
treatment for, 122–124
vitamin source, 167, 169–170, 173–174
grass. *see* plants
growth, 150, 153, 168
Gua Sha, 85–86
gums, bleeding, 172, 192. *see also* dental problems

H

Hahnemann, Samuel, 201
hair, 27, 131, 141, 169, 180
hallucinations, 171
hangovers, 194
HDL, 168
headaches. *see also* migraines
asthma, 56
breathing techniques, 204
fibromyalgia, 64, 67
foods for, 194
Liver Qi, 190
side effect of treatment, 11–12
as a symptom, 7, 15, 43, 45, 141–144
testimonials, 131, 137, 153, 155
toxicity, 93
vitamin deficiencies, 168, 170
Wind, condition of, 36
healing, slow, 172
hearing problems, 147
Heart
attacks, 180
Biotin, 172
Blood, and, 29
disease, 176, 179
enlarged, 166
Five Organ Systems, 34
foods for ailments, 191
Gua Sha, 85
problems, 169
tongue, 73
Yin Organs, 27
Heart Meridian, 24, 35, 45, 63, 186
heartbeat, irregular, 40, 45, 65, 176–177
heartburn, 44–45
Heat, condition of
arthritis, 46
asthma, 50
constipation, 57
cupping, 83
defined, 33
diarrhea, 60
Eight Principle Patterns, 31
foods for, 197
iron, 177
office visits, 72
vitamin B5, 168
vitamin C, 173
vitamin deficiencies, 170
Yang, 37
heaviness in limbs, 30
hemoglobin, 176

hemorrhoids, 181, 194
herbal medicine
  benefits and drawbacks, 198–201
  history of, 18–19
  moxabustion, 86–87
  office visits, 69
  Oriental nutrition, 182
  sensitivity treatments, 5–6
  toxicity, 93
  Traditional Chinese Medicine (TCM), 35
  treatments, 101
herbs, 122–124
hernia, hiatus, 181
hiccups, 143, 190
history of acupuncture, 18–19, 20, 21
hoarseness, 194
holistic system, 32, 35
homeopathy, 13, 20, 81, 93, 149, 201–203
homeostasis, 24, 32, 35
hormones, 28, 112–116, 124, 163, 173, 203
hot energy foods, 186
hot flashes, 44
Huang Di Nei Ching Su Wen, The, 19
hurricanes, effect on allergies, 55–56, 146
hydrochloric acid, 166, 176, 179
hyperactivity, 33
hypertension, 176–177, 180, 194
hyperthyroidism, 171
hyperventilation, 45
hypoactivity, 29
hysteria, 167

I

imbalance, defined, 33
immunizations, 153
immunoglobulins, 41
impotence, 194
incontinence, 44
indigestion, 44, 168, 194. *see also* digestive problems
infants, 179. *see also* pediatrics
infections, 165, 168
inflammation
  arthritis, 46, 48, 50
  grains, 163
  Heat, condition of, 33
  testimonials, 141
  vitamin deficiencies, 165, 167
ink, 138, 142
insects, 116–118
insomnia, 33, 44–45, 137, 165. *see also* sleep
insulin, 140–141, 163, 200
internal factors, 31, 33, 37
Internet, 199, 203
intestines, 60, 173
iron, 172, 176–177
irritability, 168, 170–171
irritable bowel syndrome, 57, 59 61, 156
itching, 12, 36, 93, 131, 143, 146–147, 167

J

jaw pain, 65
joint pain
  Dampness, condition of, 30
  as a symptom, 8–9, 15, 44
  testimonials, 131, 137
  vitamin deficiencies, 169, 172
juices, 183

K

K, vitamin, 175
keratin, 165
Kidney
  essence (jing), 32
  Five Organ Systems, 34
  foods for ailments, 191
  stones, 29, 194
  tongue, 73
  vitamin D, 174
  weakness, 194
  Yin Organs, 27
Kidney Meridian, 24, 35, 45, 53, 59, 167, 186
Kidney Qi, 26
Kidney Yang Deficiency, 60
kinesiology, 80
kissing after treatment, 92

L

lactose, 171
Large Intestine, 29, 34, 36, 57, 191
Large Intestine Meridian, 24, 58
laughter, importance of, 203
LDL, 168
leaky gut syndrome, 140
leather, 126–127
legumes, 122–124, 167–170, 175–176
lethargy, 30
Li Shi Shen, 19
ligaments, 205
light
  fibromyalgia, 64
  testimonials, 131
  treatment for, 98, 120
  vitamin D, 160, 173–174
  vitamin deficiencies, 167, 169
Liver
  Blood, and, 29
  Five Organ Systems, 34
  foods for ailments, 191
  laughter, importance of, 203
  tongue, 73
  vitamin B6, 170
  vitamin deficiencies, 166–168
  vitamin K, 175
  Yin Organs, 37
Liver Meridian, 24, 35, 45, 53, 59–60, 186
Liver Qi, 190
Lu, Henry C., 182
lumps, 34, 196
Lung Meridian
  asthma, 50, 53
  coughing, 59
  defined, 22
  digestive problems, 63

Lung Meridian *(cont.)*
Five Flavors of Food, 186
Qi, 26
Seven Emotions, 35
Lung Qi, 51, 189–190
Lung Yin Deficiency, 51
Lungs
coughing, 58–59
Five Organ Systems, 34
foods for ailments, 191
Gua Sha, 85
lubrication of, 195
tongue, 73
vitamin E, 174
Wind, condition of, 36
Yin Organs, 37
lymphatic system, 205

M

magnesium, 175–176
massage, 32
Mayo clinics, 21
medications, 124
memory loss, 166, 168, 170–171
menstruation, 44
Meridian Stress Assessment (MSA), 33, 53, 59, 132, 138, 154
Meridians. *see also* names of individual Meridians
defined, 12
defining the problem, 53, 68
Five Energies of Food, 183
Five Flavors of Food, 186
Meridians *(cont.)*
methods behind AcuSET, 30, 22–23, 24, 34, 35, 26
testimonials, 132, 135, 138–139, 141, 144
treatments, 78, 80, 87
metabolism, 171–172, 176, 180
microbial fermentation, 171
migraines, 44, 138, 144, 180. *see also* headaches
milk. *see* dairy
minerals, 100–101, 159–160, 162, 175–178
mold, 11, 98, 106–107, 145
mood swings, 65, 177
morning sickness, 195
movement of food, 189–190
moxabustion, 86–87
MRI, 78
MSA (Meridian Stress Assessment), 33, 53, 59, 132, 138, 154
MSG, 6–7, 10
mucus, 34, 193, 197–198
muscle aches, 93, 135, 166, 168, 172, 176
muscle testing, 9, 80

N

NAET (Nambudripad's Allergy Elimination Techniques), 5, 8–9, 47, 55, 134, 136–137
nails, brittle, 180
Nambudripad, Dr. Devi, 8–9

National Institutes of Health, The (NIH), 21, 202
nausea
  digestive problems, 63
  mineral deficiencies, 177
  side effect of treatment, 11
  as a symptom, 44
  testimonials, 131
  toxicity, 93
  vitamin deficiencies, 169, 172
neck pain, 10, 44, 86, 141, 145
needles, materials used for, 18
needling techniques, 19, 31, 35, 73–74, 81–83
nervous system problems, 166
neuralgia, 20
neuropathy, 166
neutral energy foods, 185
New York Times, The, 21
night blindness, 165
night sweats, 44, 65, 195
nightmares, 131
nitrogen, 178
Nixon, Richard M., 20
nodules, 30, 34
nose, runny, 40, 62, 142, 144, 147, 153
nose, stuffy, 36, 144
nosebleeds, 195
numbness, 7, 36, 65, 131, 169, 171
nutritional deficiencies, 160. *see also* deficiencies, mineral; deficiencies, vitamin
nutritional supplements. *see* supplements
nuts, 122–124, 176

O

obesity, 180–181, 207
obstructions, 34
odor, body, 24
office visits, 69–75
oils, 173–174
organ systems, defined, 34
organic food, 158–159
organ-related ailments, 191–192
Oriental nutrition, 182–190
osteomalacia, 173
osteopenia, 176
osteoporosis, 176
overeating, 44
oxidation, 158

P

pain, 27, 132–135, 195, 205
paint, 141
paleness, 27, 131
palpitations, 44–45, 135–137, 144, 170
panic attacks as a symptom. *see* anxiety
paper, sensitivity to, 138, 142
pathogens, 34
pathology, 19
paying before treatment, 92
pediatrics, 14–15, 149–156
pellagra, 160, 168

perfume, 14, 54–55, 57, 91–93, 99, 141
Pericardium Meridian, 22
perspiration, 194
pesticides, 116–118, 158
pets, sensitivity to, 11, 14, 52, 95, 147–149, 151
phenolics, treatment for, 96–97
phlegm
  asthma, 53, 57
  cold, condition of, 29
  coughing, 59
  Dampness, condition of, 30
  defined, 34
  Excess, 31
  Five Energies of Food, 184
  foods for, 197–198
  testimonials, 147, 152
phosphorous, 173
physiology, 19
planning for treatment, 90–93
plantar fascitis, 64
plants, 11, 14, 55–56, 109–112, 141, 145, 155
PMS, 44
pneumonia, 53–54
pollen. *see* plants
pollution, 174
polyps, 181
potassium, 177–178
poultry, 102, 168–169, 177
preeclampsia, 176
pregnancy, 72, 87, 170–171, 174, 177
processed foods, 188, 207
proteins, 168–170, 172, 178–180, 181, 200
prothrombin, 175
psoriasis, 180
puffiness of eyes or nose, 39–40
pulse, slow, 166
pulse positions, 19, 24, 70–71, 73
pungent flavors, 187

Q

Qi
  defining the problem, 46, 63
  Five Energies of Food, 183
  Five Flavors of Food, 189
  foods for, 198
  methods behind AcuSET, 29, 30, 31–32, 33, 34, 37
  movement of food, 189–190
  office visits, 70–71
  treatments, 82–83, 85, 87
  vitamins, 168, 171

R

radiation, 78, 120, 155
rashes, skin
  fibromyalgia, 65, 67
  foods for, 196
  Heat, condition of, 33
  as a symptom, 15, 44, 145–147
  testimonials, 131, 137, 143, 150, 153–155
  vitamin deficiencies, 169, 172
RDA, 161, 174

redness, 147, 167
reflexology, 32
Ren Meridian, 24, 23
Rescue Remedy, 202–203
respiratory problems, 153
restless leg syndrome, 65
restlessness, 33, 36
Reston, James, 21
rheumatism, 20
Rhijne, Willem Ten, 20
rickets, 160, 173
ringing in ears, 131
RNA, 162
runny nose, 15, 40, 62, 142, 144, 147, 153

S

salt, 41, 121, 138
salty flavors, 187, 190
School of Complementary Medicine, 5
sedation, 34
sensitivity elimination treatments, 90
Seven Emotions, 35
shakiness, 45
Shands, 21
shoulder pain, 141
sinusitis
  breathing techniques, 204
  diarrhea, 62
  fibromyalgia, 67
  foods for, 196
  pressure, 56–58
  as a symptom, 144–145
sinusitis *(cont.)*
  testimonials, 133, 137, 143, 150, 152–153
skin color, 17, 23, 69–70
skin problems, 36, 65, 131, 180
sleep. *see also* fatigue; insomnia
  anxiety, 46
  balance, importance of, 24
  caffeine, 189
  fibromyalgia, 64
  nutritional deficiencies, 160
  testimonials, 133–134, 141, 144, 153, 157
  vitamin deficiencies, 168
  vitamins, 165
Small Intestine, 34, 36, 192
Small Intestine Meridian, 22
smell, 54–55, 64, 147
smog, 174
smoke, 11, 57–58, 71, 119, 157
sneezing
  asthma, 50
  diarrhea, 62
  side effect of treatment, 12
  as a symptom, 15, 40, 147–150
  testimonials, 131
  Wind, condition of, 36
snoring, 14
sodium, 177
sores, 147, 168, 172
sound, 64, 131, 169
sour flavors, 187, 190
soy, 96, 112–116, 145–146, 169, 171

spasms, 29, 36, 169, 176
spices, 122–124
spirit (shen), 35
Spleen
  Blood, and, 29
  Five Organ Systems, 34
  foods for ailments, 192
  Gua Sha, 85
  tongue, 73
  vitamin B5, 168
  vitamin deficiencies, 166
  Yin Organs, 37
Spleen Meridian, 24, 35, 53, 60, 62, 183, 186–188
Spleen Qi, 45
Spleen Yang Deficiency, 60
stabbing pain, 184
stagnation, 30, 31, 33, 35, 26, 85–87, 197
stiffness, joint, 46, 169
Stomach, 34, 36, 73, 168, 170, 183, 192
Stomach Meridian, 24, 35, 59, 62, 167, 186–187
Stomach Qi, 189
Stomach Yin Deficiency, 63
stomachaches, 155, 196
stools, problems with, 29, 30, 156, 189
stress, 145, 147, 168, 203, 205. *see also* anxiety
strokes, 180
stuffy nose, 36, 144
sugar, 46, 119, 163–164, 166, 168, 180
Sun Si-miao, 182
sunscreen, 174
supplements, 65, 158–165
surgery, 205
sweats, night, 44, 65, 195
sweet flavors, 188, 190
swelling, 30, 33, 50, 65, 131, 145–146
symptoms, foods to correct, 196–198
symptoms of sensitivities, 43–67

T

Tang dynasty, 182
TCM (Traditional Chinese Medicine), 35
techniques, needling, 35, 81–83
tendons, 205
tension release techniques, 203–204
testimonials
  anxiety, 137–138
  asthma, 52–55, 151
  coughing, 143–144
  diarrhea, 60–64
  digestive problems, 140–141
  fibromyalgia, 66–67, 138–140
  headaches, 141–143
  hearing problems, 147
  multiple symptoms, 131–132
  pain, 132–135
  palpitations, 135–137
  pediatrics, 149–156
  rashes, skin, 145–147

testimonials *(cont.)*
  sinusitis, 144–145
  sneezing, 147–149
testosterone, 168
thirst, relief of, 195
thought, cloudiness of, 134, 166
throat problems, 36, 44, 51, 141, 196
Thyroid Gland Meridian, 53
tingling, 65, 166, 169, 171
tongue, diagnosis by looking at, 72–73, 132–133
tongue, sore, 170
tonify, defined, 35
toothaches. *see* dental problems
toxins, 173, 205
Traditional Chinese Medicine (TCM), 35
trans fats, 179
trauma, 30
treatments
  afterwards, 127–128
  alcohol, 126
  amino acids, 93–94
  animals, 95
  caffeine and leather, 126
  chemicals and cleaners, 121
  corn, grains, spices, nuts, legumes and herbs, 122–124
  detoxifying, 93
  dust and mold, 106–107
  eating, timing of, 89–92
  eating before treatment, 121
  eggs and poultry, 102
treatments *(cont.)*
  environmentals, 98–99
  fish, 125–126
  food additives, 107–108
  fuels, 102
  hormones and fats, 112–116
  insects and pesticides, 116–118
  medications and vaccinations, 124
  minerals, 100–101
  overview of, 77–87
  phenolics, 96–97
  planning for, 90–93
  plants, 109–112
  radiation, 120
  salt, 121
  smoke, 119
  sugar, 119
  vitamin B, 118
  vitamin C, fruits, vegetables and vinegar, 103–105
trees. *see* plants
trembling, 36
tremors, 176
Triple Burner Qi, 190
Triple Warmer Meridian, 22
tumors, 34, 196

U

ulcerative colitis, 59
University of Florida, Gainesville, 21
urinary tract infections, 29
urination, problems with, 33, 131, 195

V

vaccinations, 124
varicose veins, 181
vegetarians, 174
vertigo. *see* dizziness
vials, 75, 81
vinegar, 103–105
viruses, 34, 41, 59, 67
vision, blurred, 65, 138, 147
visits, office, 69–75
vitamins. *see also* names of individual vitamins
- anxiety, 46
- information about, 158–162
- supplements, 164–175
- testimonials, 157
- treatment for, 103–105, 112–116, 118, 125–127

voice, weak, 50, 133
vomiting, 7, 44–45, 63, 131, 189–190, 196

W

warm energy foods, 185–186
watery eyes, 147–148
weakness, 27, 133–135, 166, 170, 176–177
weeds. *see* plants
weight gain, 145, 150, 187, 207
weight loss, 170, 173
wheezing, 50, 54, 144
Wind, condition of, 24, 31, 36, 46, 50, 83
Winfrey, Oprah, 21
wool, 10

X

X-rays, 54, 78, 120

Y

Yang, 19, 27, 28, 31, 46, 174–176, 198
Yang Organs, 36
Yang Qi, 198
yawning, 131
Yin, 19, 28, 31, 36–37, 46, 189, 198
Yin Organs, 37
YinTang, 203

www.debragaffney.com